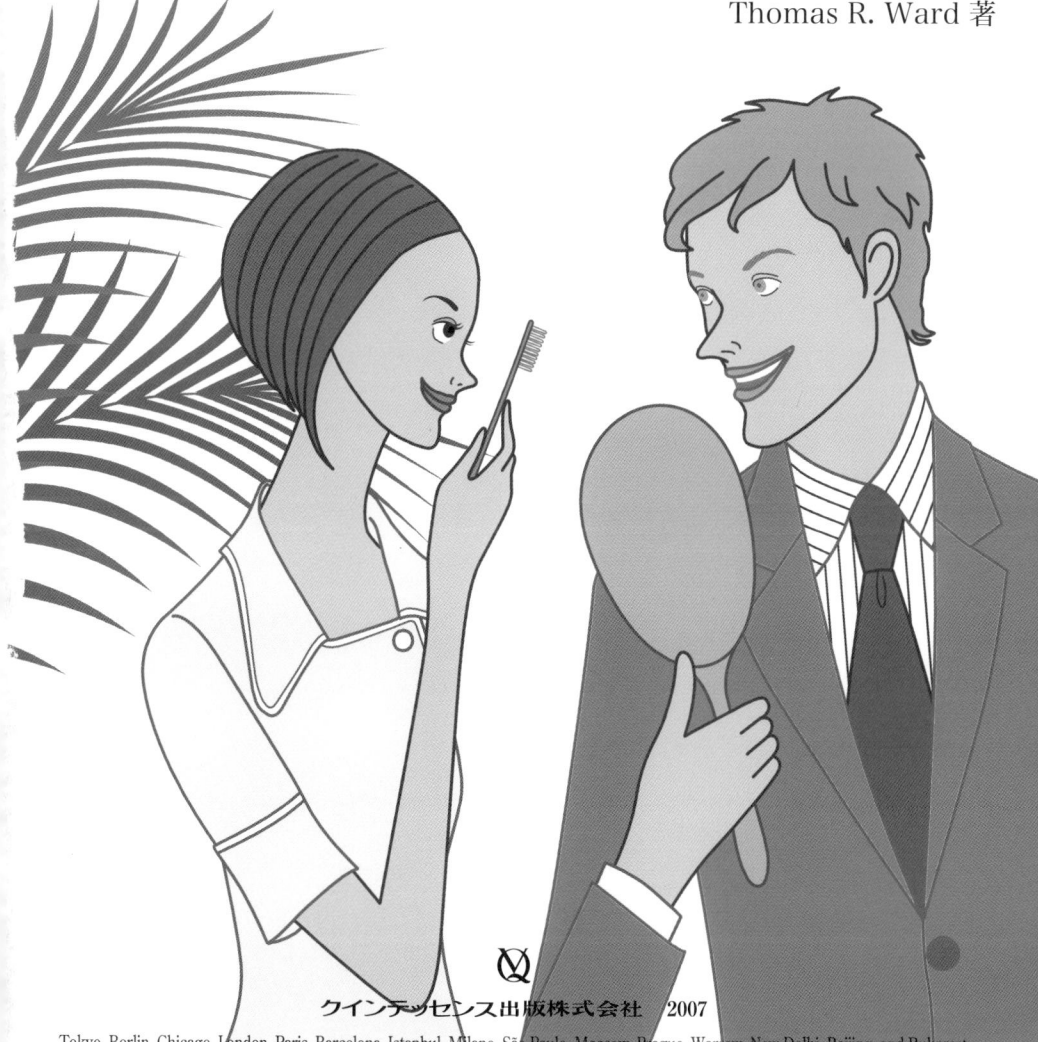

まえがき

　この本は、歯科衛生士やアシスタントが外国人患者とコミュニケーションするうえで、手助けになるように書かれた2冊のうちの第1冊目である。現在、日本には200万人以上の外国人が在住している。そしてさらに、毎年700万人を越える人々が日本を訪れている。こうした傾向は日本の国際化により、今後ますます増えていくであろう。この外国人たちは、開発途上国からの留学生、教師、ビジネスマン、外交官など、さまざまな職業や国籍の人々である。

　歯科衛生士やアシスタントと外国人患者のコミュニケーションでは、いろいろな問題が起こりかねない。一般的に言って外国人は、日本人に比べて自分の受ける治療の説明を求めることが多いようである。また、国や職業の違いのため、患者が歯科治療に何を期待しているか、はっきりとつかみにくいこともある。コミュニケーションは、子どもを扱うときに、特に重要なポイントになる。この本では、歯科衛生士やアシスタントが日常の診療で、外国人患者と話すときに役立つような、基本的会話を集めた。

　本書をマスターすることによって、外国人患者にも積極的に歯科衛生士やアシスタントの方々が接していくことを期待する。

Thomas R. Ward

本書の使用にあたって

　本書は、独学にも、また教室での勉強にも使用できる。歯科診療で外国人患者と接する際の日常的なシチュエーションで、口腔清掃の必要性や歯ブラシ指導、フッ化物などのいろいろな説明を、基本的な会話の形で集めたものである。

　本書は10章からなり、それぞれ2つのセクションに分かれている。最初は歯科の1つのトピックを患者にもわかる平易な表現で説明する対話になっている。この対話では専門用語は使っていない。各章の対話の前には、場面の説明を簡単にしているが、この中には、歯科医や歯科衛生士だけが使う専門用語が含まれていることもある。

　第2のセクションは、対話中の文章を使った5つの入れ換え練習問題がある。ここに使われている用語は、専門的な性格のもの（う蝕原性の、歯肉切除術など）、患者が理解できる言葉（むし歯、クラウンなど）もある。この問題は、マスターするまで反復練習をするとよいだろう。

　本書の最後には、歯科衛生士と患者のコミュニケーションのための、もっとも重要な100語を載せた。これらは、歯科用語を特に知らない人にでもわかる言葉である。このような言葉は、患者とのコミュニケーションに欠かせないものなので、対話の勉強を始める前に暗記するのも良いだろう。

　独学の方には、収録した音声が大変役に立つことと思う。

CD（収録音声）の使い方

　本書とセットになったCDには、次のものが収録されている。①各章の英会話すべて、②各章の練習問題の例題すべて、③各章の練習問題の置き換え語句すべて。

１．各章の英会話を練習する順序と方法
①まず、会話全体をとおして聞いてみる。
②発音と意味がわかったところで、実際に声を出して会話を模倣する。この際、１人が話す度ごとに音声を止め、反復練習をしてみると効果的である。
③次に、自分が対話の一方の役になって、その部分を言ってみる。たとえば、登場している歯科衛生士になったつもりで、患者の発音ごとに音声を止め、歯科衛生士の応答文を言ってみる。次いで音声を再開し、自分の発音、イントネーションが正しいかどうか確認する。この役割練習は、歯科衛生士だけでなく、患者にもなって行うべきである。
④次に双方の役割を１人でこなして、全文を暗記してみる。この際、会話にあるイントネーションを意識的にまねてみることが重要である。

２．練習問題の使い方
①例題と語句の置き換わったものを２〜３回聞き、声を出して反復練習してみる。
②発音とイントネーションを耳と口が覚えたと思ったら、練習問題の置き換え語句を入れ換えて、次々声を出して練習してみる。
③その際、１つずつ置き換え語句ごとに音声を止め、声を出して置き換えられた文を発音してみる。
④置き換え文章を12まで発音し終わったら、また１まで戻り、置き換えがスムーズに言えるようにする。
⑤置き換えがスムーズに言えるようになったら、自分で置き換え語句を考え出し、どんどん置き換え文を作ってみる。自分の毎日の仕事と職場を想定し、どんどん楽しい置き換え文を作ってみよう。

　以上、短時間でも繰り返し行ってみよう。英会話の習得は、納得のいくまで声を出して練習することがコツである。

CONTENTS

まえがき ……………………………………………………… 3

本書の使用にあたって ………………………………… 4

CD（収録音声）の使い方 …………………………… 5

第1章　歯科衛生士の処置を患者に説明する 　　　　Ⅰ．なぜ口腔清掃が必要か ……………… 8 　Why Do I Need to Have My Teeth Cleaned? 　どうして私の歯をクリーニングしてもらわなくちゃいけないんですか？

第2章　歯科衛生士の処置を患者に説明する 　　　　Ⅱ．口腔清掃はどういうものか ………… 22 　How Can I Talk When You Have Your Hands in My Mouth? 　あなたの手が口の中に入っているのに、どうやって話したらいいのですか？

第3章　歯科衛生士の処置を患者に説明する 　　　　Ⅲ．再来院が必要な患者の2度目の治療 ……… 36 　I Might be Here a Long Time. 　ここに長期間来ることになるかもしれませんね

第4章　歯科衛生士の処置を患者に説明する 　　　　Ⅳ．口腔清掃の仕上げ …………………… 50 　The Gums Are Still Red and Puffed Up. 　歯ぐきがまだ赤くて腫れています

第5章　小さな子どもが初めて歯科衛生士と接する時
Ⅰ．何をするか説明する ……………………… 62
You're Not So Bad After All.
お姉さんもそんなに悪くないね

第6章　小さな子どもが初めて歯科衛生士と接する時
Ⅱ．器具や設備の説明 ……………………… 76
Sometimes Sugar Bugs Hide Between the Teeth.
時々、砂糖の虫は歯と歯の間に隠れているの

第7章　小さな子どもが初めて歯科衛生士と接する時
Ⅲ．歯ブラシ指導 ……………………… 90
What Are Sugar Bugs?
砂糖の虫って何？

第8章　小さな子どもが初めて歯科衛生士と接する時
Ⅳ．フロッシング指導 ……………………… 104
Those Sugar Bugs Were Hiding Everywhere.
その砂糖の虫はいろんなところに隠れていたんだね

第9章　小さな子どもが初めて歯科衛生士と接する時
Ⅴ．フッ素の応用 ……………………… 116
What is Fluoride?
フッ素って何？

第10章　既往歴 ……………………… 128
Are You in Good Health?
健康状態はよいですか？

付録 ……………………… 140
患者とのコミュニケーションで役立つ最重要用語100語

Chapter 1

An explanation of the hygienist's treatment
Part I: Why oral prophylaxis is necessary

Why Do I Need to Have My Teeth Cleaned?

The foreigners in Japan come from a wide variety of backgrounds. Some may visit the dentist every six months for an examination and oral prophylaxis; these people will be very familiar with the need for an oral prophylaxis. Others may go to the dentist only when they have a toothache. This type of person may not have a clear idea what the hygienist does or why an oral prophylaxis is necessary. Sometimes it may be necessary for the hygienist to explain to the patient why this treatment is necessary.

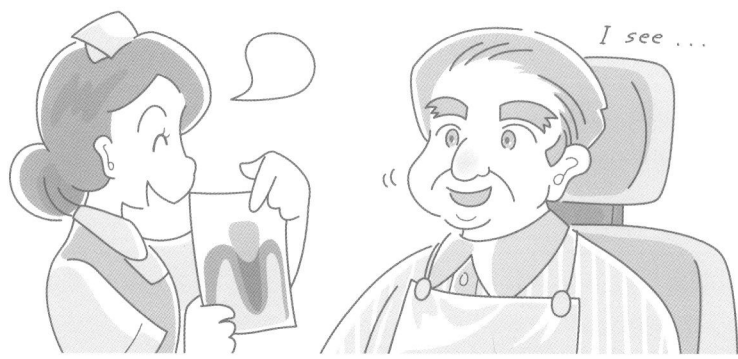

第 1 章

歯科衛生士の処置を患者に説明する
Ⅰ．なぜ口腔清掃が必要か

どうして私の歯をクリーニングしてもらわなくちゃいけないんですか？

　日本にいる外国人は、さまざまな経歴を持っている。検査と口腔清掃のため6ヵ月ごとに歯医者に行く人たちもいる。この人たちは、口腔清掃の必要性を大変よく知っている。その他の人は、歯痛があるときだけ歯医者に行くという人たちかもしれない。こういうタイプの人は、歯科衛生士の仕事や、なぜ口腔清掃が必要かはっきりわかっていないことがある。時には、なぜその治療が必要なのか、歯科衛生士が患者に説明しなければならない。

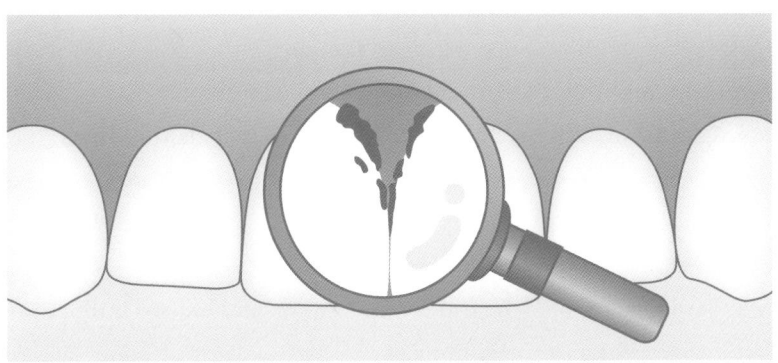

Situation: Mr. Rupert, age 49, came to the dental clinic because of gingival bleeding and pain. This is his first visit to the dentist in 20 years. The dentist has informed him that he has an advanced periodontal condition and that a thorough cleaning will be necessary before the examination can be completed.

Ms. Terasaki (dental hygienist): Would you please come in here, Mr. Rupert?

Mr. Rupert: Certainly, I'll be glad to. Are you a dentist?

Ms. Terasaki: No, I am a dental hygienist. Dr. Wada has asked me to clean your teeth before he continues with the examination and diagnosis.

Mr. Rupert: Why do I need to have my teeth cleaned? I can clean them myself. I have a toothbrush right here.

Ms. Terasaki: A toothbrush is not adequate to remove the deposits and stains on your teeth. Here look in this mirror. (She gives him a hand mirror, turns on the chair light, and places the mouth mirror behind his mandibular anterior teeth.)

Mr. Rupert: What's that yellow stuff on my teeth?

Ms. Terasaki: That is calculus. It is mainly calcium from the saliva which has formed hard deposits on the teeth.

Mr. Rupert: It sure looks ugly.

Ms. Terasaki: It also irritates the gums and is an important factor in gum disease.

場面：49歳のルパート氏は、歯肉出血と痛みのために来院。この20年間歯医者に行ったことがない。歯科医は、彼の歯周状態が悪化しているので診査を終える前に徹底的なクリーニングが必要だと告げた。

寺崎さん（歯科衛生士）：ルパートさん、こちらにお入りになってくださいますか？
ルパート氏：ええ、もちろんですとも。あなたが歯医者さんですか？
　寺崎：いいえ、私は歯科衛生士です。和田先生から、診査と診断を続ける前にルパートさんの歯をクリーニングするように言われましたので。
ルパート氏：どうしてクリーニングしてもらわなくちゃいけないんですか？　自分でできますよ。ここに歯ブラシもあります。
　寺崎：歯ブラシだけでは、歯の付着物やしみを取り除くのに十分ではないのです。ほら、この鏡をご覧になってください。（手鏡を渡し、診療椅子のあかりを付け、ミラーを彼の下顎前歯の後ろに当てる。）

ルパート氏：歯についている黄色いのは何ですか？
　寺崎：それは歯石です。主に唾液のカルシウムが歯の上で固い付着物となったものです。

ルパート氏：本当に汚く見えますね。
　寺崎：それは歯ぐきを刺激もしますし、歯ぐきの病気の重要な要因になります。

Mr. Rupert: I guess I should brush more often.

Ms. Terasaki: Brushing alone will not remove calculus. You should visit a dentist at least once every six months and have your teeth cleaned by a dental hygienist.

Mr. Rupert: I guess you're right.

ルパート氏：もっとよく磨いた方がよさそうですね。

寺崎：ブラッシングだけでは歯石は取れないんです。少なくとも6ヵ月に1度歯医者に行って、歯科衛生士に歯をクリーニングしてもらわなければなりません。

ルパート氏：そのようですね。

Exercises

Ⅰ. Substitute the following expressions in the example sentence.

Some people brush their teeth three times a day.
〈twice a day〉
Some people brush their teeth twice a day.

  1. four times a day
  2. every day
  3. frequently
  4. when they have a date
  5. before they go to the dentist
  6. every week
  7. when their dentist tells them to brush
  8. once in a while
  9. every hour
  10. when they get gum disease
  11. when they get a toothache
  12. when they remember

Ⅱ. Substitute the following expressions in the example sentence.

The dentist has informed him that he has an advanced periodontal condition.
〈gum disease〉
The dentist has informed him that he has gum disease.

練習問題

Ⅰ．例文の下線部を以下の語句に置き換えなさい。

1日に3回歯を磨く人たちもいる。
〈1日に2回〉
1日に2回歯を磨く人たちもいる。

1. 1日に4回
2. 毎日
3. しばしば
4. デートがある時
5. 歯医者に行く前に
6. 毎週
7. 歯医者に磨くように言われた時
8. たまに
9. 毎時間
10. 歯ぐきの病気になった時
11. 歯痛になった時
12. 思い出したら

Ⅱ．例文の下線部を以下の語句に置き換えなさい。

歯科医は、彼に悪化している歯周状態があると告げた。

〈歯ぐきの病気〉
歯科医は、彼に歯ぐきの病気があると告げた。

1. periodontal disease
2. oral hygiene problems
3. bad breath
4. need for treatment
5. mild gingivitis
6. minimal dental needs
7. an oral cancer
8. no problems
9. calculus deposits
10. decay
11. an enlarged tongue
12. malocclusion

Ⅲ. Substitute the following expressions in the example dialogue.

－Would you please come in here?
－Certainly, I'll be glad to.
〈brush your teeth〉
－Would you please brush your teeth?
－Certainly, I'll be glad to.

1. rinse your mouth
2. ask the dentist
3. floss every day
4. remove the calculus
5. polish the teeth
6. remove the coffee stains

1. 歯周病がある
2. 口腔衛生の問題がある
3. 口臭がある
4. 治療の必要性がある
5. 軽い歯肉炎がある
6. 治療を必要とする所は少ない
7. 口腔癌がある
8. 問題が何もない
9. 歯石沈着物がある
10. むし歯がある
11. 肥大した舌がある
12. 不正咬合がある

Ⅲ．例にあげた対話の下線部を以下の語句に置き換えなさい。

－<u>こちらにお入りになって</u>くださいますか？
－ええ。もちろんですとも。
〈あなたの歯を磨く〉
－あなたの歯を磨いてくださいますか？
－ええ。もちろんですとも。

1. あなたの口をゆすぐ
2. 歯医者に聞く
3. 毎日フロッシングする
4. 歯石を除去する
5. 歯を研磨する
6. コーヒーのしみを除去する

7. see the hygienist
8. give the patient oral hygiene instructions
9. brush the patient's teeth
10. treat the gum disease
11. buy a new toothbrush
12. use floss every day

Ⅳ. Substitute the following expressions in the example sentence.

I guess I should <u>brush</u> more often.
〈floss〉
I guess I should <u>floss</u> more often.

1. see the dentist
2. have my teeth cleaned
3. brush my teeth
4. have my teeth polished
5. floss my teeth
6. have the hygienist clean my teeth
7. see the hygienist
8. have cleaning appointments
9. have checkups
10. brush and floss my teeth
11. have my gums checked
12. have dental appointments

7. 歯科衛生士に診てもらう
8. 患者に口腔衛生指導をする
9. 患者の歯を磨く
10. 歯ぐきの病気を治療する
11. 新しい歯ブラシを買う
12. 毎日フロッシングする

Ⅳ．例文の下線部を以下の語句に置き換えなさい。

もっとよく磨いた方がよさそうですね。
〈フロスする〉
もっとよくフロスした方がよさそうですね。

1. 歯科医を訪れる
2. 歯をクリーニングしてもらう
3. 私の歯を磨く
4. 私の歯を研磨してもらう
5. 私の歯をフロスする
6. 歯科衛生士に歯をきれいにしてもらう
7. 歯科衛生士に診てもらう
8. クリーニングのためのアポイントをとる
9. 検診を受ける
10. 私の歯を磨いてフロスする
11. 私の歯ぐきをチェックしてもらう
12. 歯科のアポイントをとる

V. Substitute the following expressions in the example sentence.

Plaque is an important factor in gum disease.
⟨periodontal disease⟩
Plaque is an important factor in periodontal disease.

1. bad breath
2. tooth decay
3. dental caries
4. halitosis
5. calculus formation
6. oral health
7. gingival health
8. acid production
9. bleeding gums
10. gingival pocket formation
11. dental disease
12. gingivitis

Ⅴ．例文の下線部を以下の語句に置き換えなさい。

プラークは歯ぐきの病気の重要な要因になります。
〈歯周病〉
プラークは歯周病の重要な要因になります。

1. 口臭
2. むし歯
3. う蝕
4. 口臭
5. 歯石の形成
6. 口腔の健康
7. 歯ぐきの健康
8. 酸が生じること
9. 歯ぐきの出血
10. 歯周ポケットの形成
11. 歯科疾患
12. 歯肉炎

Chapter 2

An explanation of the hygienist's treatment
Part II: What oral prophylaxis involves

How Can I Talk When You Have Your Hands in My Mouth?

Explain to your patients what you are going to do. Many of them may already know what a hygienist does and some others may not know anything. Your explanation should conform to the needs of the patient. Be sure to ask, "Do you have any questions?"

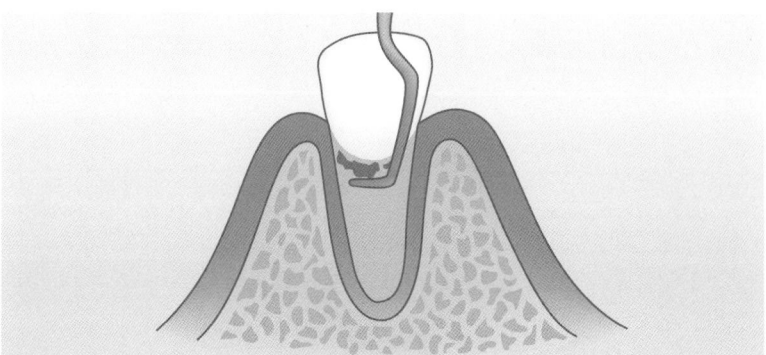

第 2 章

歯科衛生士の処置を患者に説明する
Ⅱ．口腔清掃はどういうものか

あなたの手が口の中に入っているのに、どうやって話したらいいのですか？

　あなたがすることを患者に説明すること。多くの人は歯科衛生士が何をするか知っているが、何も知らない人もいる。説明は、患者のニーズに応じてすること。必ず、「何か質問がありますか」と尋ねなければならない。

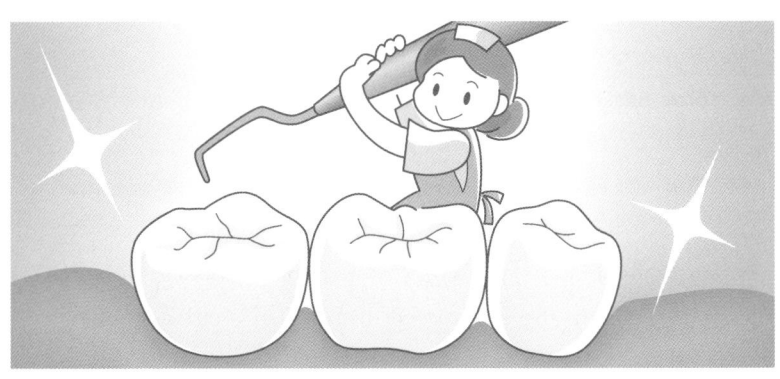

Situation: A continuation of the previous dialogue. The hygienist is about to begin cleaning Mr. Rupert's teeth.

Ms. Terasaki (dental hygienist): Do you have any questions about this treatment?
Mr. Rupert: How will you get that calculus off my teeth?
Ms. Terasaki: First, I will use this ultrasonic scaler. It makes a buzzing noise, sprays a mist of water, and breaks up the calculus and plaque.
Mr. Rupert: Does it hurt?
Ms. Terasaki: The teeth may be a bit sensitive. If it feels uncomfortable, tell me and I will stop.
Mr. Rupert: How can I talk when you have your hands in my mouth?
Ms. Terasaki: It is not necessary to talk. If you feel uncomfortable, just raise your hand and let me know.
Mr. Rupert: O.K., I will.
Ms. Terasaki: After the deposits have been removed using the ultrasonic scaler, I will use these scalers to clean between the teeth and remove the remaining calculus.
Mr. Rupert: That thing looks like it might hurt.
Ms. Terasaki: You will feel the scraping but it should not be too uncomfortable.
Mr. Rupert: How about the black stain? Can you get that off, too?
Ms. Terasaki: That is probably stain from coffee or tobacco. It can be removed using this rubber cup and handpiece.

場面：前章の対話の続き。歯科衛生士がルパート氏の歯のクリーニングを始めようとしている。

寺崎さん（歯科衛生士）：この治療について何かご質問はありますか？
ルパート氏：どのようにして歯から歯石を取るんですか？
　　寺崎：最初に、この超音波スケーラーを使います。ブーンという音を立てて、霧状の水を噴射し、歯石やプラークを壊していくわけです。
ルパート氏：痛いですか？
　　寺崎：歯が少し過敏になるかもしれません。もし痛いときは、おっしゃってくだされば止めます。
ルパート氏：あなたの手が口の中に入っているのに、どうやって話したらいいのですか？
　　寺崎：話す必要はありません。もし痛ければ、ちょっと手を上げて知らせてください。
ルパート氏：わかりました。そうしましょう。
　　寺崎：超音波スケーラーを使って付着物を取り除いた後、このスケーラーを使って歯と歯の間をきれいにし、残っている歯石を除去します。

ルパート氏：それは痛そうに見えますね。
　　寺崎：削っているのは感じられるでしょうが、そんなに痛いものではありません。
ルパート氏：黒いしみはどうするのですか？　それも取れるんですか？
　　寺崎：それは多分、コーヒーかたばこのしみでしょう。このラバーカップとハンドピースを使えば取れます。

Mr. Rupert: How long will this take?
Ms. Terasaki: It will probably take two appointments of about forty-five minutes each.
Mr. Rupert: That's a lot of time.
Ms. Terasaki: Your teeth are important. We must get them clean before the dentist can continue the treatment.
Mr. Rupert: I agree.

ルパート氏：どのくらい時間がかかりますか？
　　寺崎：たぶん、45分ずつ2回のアポイントがかかるでしょう。

ルパート氏：長いですね。
　　寺崎：歯は大切ですから。歯医者が治療を続ける前に、歯をきれいにしなければなりません。
ルパート氏：そうですね。

Exercises

I. Substitute the following expressions in the example sentence.

He does not even know <u>what a dental hygienist does</u>.
〈what a dentist does〉
He does not even know <u>what a dentist does</u>.

1. what a filling is
2. what a toothbrush is
3. how to hold a toothbrush
4. how to hold the floss
5. how to brush his teeth
6. how to take care of his teeth
7. what a crown is
8. what periodontal disease is
9. what plaque is
10. what calculus is
11. what floss looks like
12. how many teeth he has

II. Substitute the following expressions in the example sentence.

Do you have any questions about <u>this treatment</u>?
〈dentistry〉
Do you have any questions about <u>dentistry</u>?

練習問題

Ⅰ．例文の下線部を以下の語句に置き換えなさい。

彼は、歯科衛生士が何をするかを知りもしない。
〈歯科医が何をするか〉
彼は、歯科医が何をするかを知りもしない。

1. 充填物とは何か
2. 歯ブラシとは何か
3. 歯ブラシの持ち方
4. フロスの持ち方
5. 歯の磨き方
6. 歯のケアの仕方
7. クラウンとは何か
8. 歯周病とは何か
9. プラークとは何か
10. 歯石とは何か
11. フロスはどのように見えるか
12. 自分は歯が何本あるか

Ⅱ．例文の下線部を以下の語句に置き換えなさい。

この治療について何かご質問はありますか？
〈歯科医学〉
歯科医学について何かご質問はありますか？

1. this dental treatment
2. oral hygiene
3. cleaning
4. how to treat gum disease
5. home dental care
6. the need for treatment
7. your dental health
8. your teeth
9. the treatment plan
10. plaque
11. flossing
12. dental floss

Ⅲ. Substitute the following expressions in the example sentence.

How can I <u>talk</u> when you have your hands in my mouth?

〈think〉
How can I <u>think</u> when you have your hands in my mouth?

1. say anything
2. concentrate
3. brush
4. do anything
5. floss
6. listen

1. この歯科治療
2. 口腔衛生
3. クリーニング
4. 歯ぐきの病気の治療の仕方
5. 家庭での歯のケア
6. 治療の必要性
7. あなたの歯の健康
8. あなたの歯
9. 治療計画
10. プラーク
11. フロッシング
12. デンタルフロス

Ⅲ．例文の下線部を以下の語句に置き換えなさい。

あなたの手が口の中に入っているのに、どうやって<u>話し</u>たらいいのですか？
〈考える〉
あなたの手が口の中に入っているのに、どうやって<u>考え</u>たらいいのですか？

1. 何か言う
2. 集中する
3. 磨く
4. 何かする
5. フロスする
6. 聞く

7. think about dental health

8. think about brushing

9. think about plaque

10. ask a question

11. talk to you

12. look at you

Ⅳ. Substitute the following expressions in the example sentence.

That thing looks like it might <u>hurt</u>.
⟨be a scaler⟩
That thing looks like it might <u>be a scaler</u>.

1. sting

2. taste bad

3. cause tooth decay

4. hurt my teeth

5. clean my teeth

6. hurt my gums

7. be uncomfortable

8. cause sensitivity

9. be difficult to use

10. be easy to use

11. remove calculus

12. cause problems

7．歯の健康について考える
8．ブラッシングについて考える
9．プラークについて考える
10．質問する
11．あなたと話す
12．あなたを見る

Ⅳ．例文の下線部を以下の語句に置き換えなさい。

それは痛そうに見えますね。
〈スケーラー〉
それはスケーラーのように見えますね。

1．ちくっとする
2．まずい
3．むし歯の原因になる
4．歯を傷つける
5．歯がきれいになる
6．歯ぐきを傷つける
7．気持ちが悪い
8．過敏の原因になる
9．使うのが難しい
10．使うのが簡単だ
11．歯石を除去する
12．問題の原因になる

V. Substitute the following expressions in the example dialogue.

- How long will it take to clean my teeth?
- It will probably take two appointments of forty-five minutes each. ⟨two, forty-five minute appointments⟩
- How long will it take to clean my teeth?
- It will probably take two, forty-five minute appointments.

1. two appointments
2. one, thirty minute appointment
3. two or three appointments
4. twenty minutes
5. a short time
6. about ten minutes
7. approximately ten minutes
8. a few minutes
9. a long time
10. ten minutes for the polish only
11. a few more minutes
12. a little time

Ⅴ．例にあげた対話の下線部を以下の語句に置き換えなさい。

－私の歯をクリーニングするのにどのくらい時間がかかりますか？
－たぶん、45分ずつ2回のアポイントがかかるでしょう。
〈45分のアポイントが2回〉
－私の歯をクリーニングするのにどのくらい時間がかかりますか？
－たぶん、45分のアポイントが2回かかるでしょう。

1. 2回のアポイント
2. 30分のアポイントが1回
3. 2～3回のアポイント
4. 20分
5. 短い時間
6. だいたい10分
7. 約10分
8. 2～3分
9. 長い時間
10. 研磨だけのために10分
11. あと2～3分
12. 少しの間

Chapter 3

An explanation of the hygienist's treatment
Part III: The second appointment for a patient requiring two visits with the hygienist

I Might be Here a Long Time.

When a patient returns to have his oral prophylaxis finished, ask him if his gingival condition has improved and if there are any areas of tenderness remaining from the previous appointment. He will be happy that you are interested in his health. Also, it is important to know if there are any problem areas which are causing sensitivity. People who had a large amount of calculus before their first appointment will usually feel considerably better after the treatment. Often they will thank the hygienist.

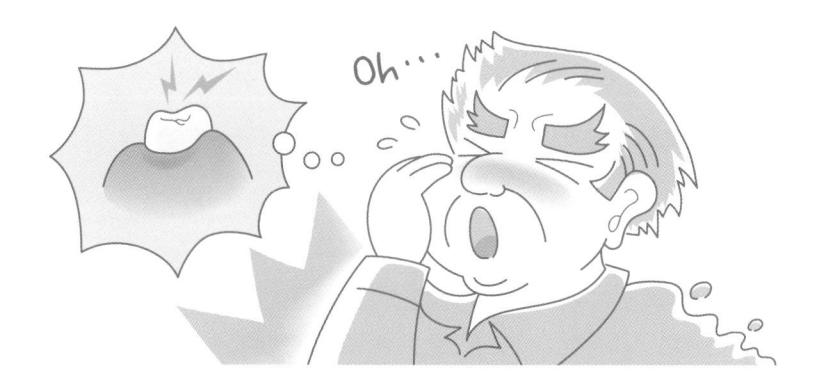

第 3 章

歯科衛生士の処置を患者に説明する
Ⅲ．再来院が必要な患者の2度目の治療

ここに長期間来ることになるかもしれませんね

　患者が口腔清掃を終えるために再来院するときは、歯肉の状態が良くなったかどうか、また、前のアポイントからどこか痛いところが残っているかどうか尋ねることである。患者は、自分の健康に興味を示されたことで喜ぶであろう。また、過敏になっているような問題の場所があるかどうか知ることも大切である。1回目のアポイントの前に歯石がたくさんあった人は、治療の後、前より気持ちよく感じるのが普通である。彼らは、歯科衛生士に感謝をすることが多い。

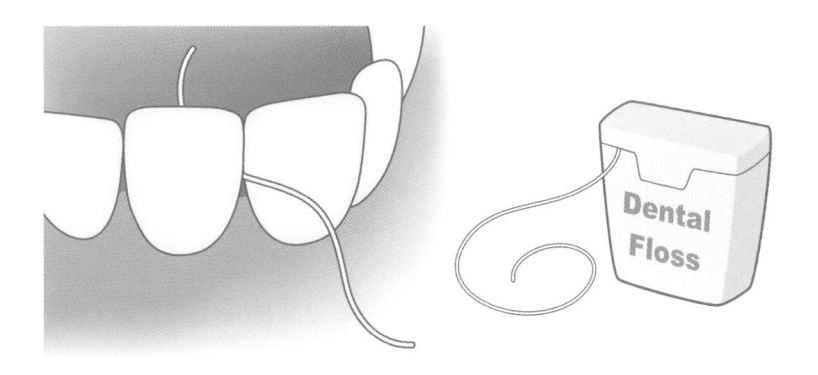

Situation: A continuation of the previous dialogue. Mr. Rupert is returning to have the oral prophylaxis completed.

Ms. Terasaki: How did your gums feel after the last appointment?

Mr. Rupert: They felt much better. They used to bleed whenever I ate an apple. Now there is no bleeding.

Ms. Terasaki: That's good. Are there any tender areas?

Mr. Rupert: The lower right in the back is a bit sensitive to cold.
Ms. Terasaki: That often happens when we clean the teeth. The sensitivity should go away in a few weeks.
Mr. Rupert: Will my gum disease be cured today?
Ms. Terasaki: No, that will take a long time and require a lot of effort on your part. You have to learn how to brush, floss, and take care of your teeth every day.

Mr. Rupert: But will you finish the cleaning today?

Ms. Terasaki: I will finish but the dentist will have to do a deep pocket cleaning. This involves getting the calculus out of the deeper pockets and it may be necessary to do gum surgery.

Mr. Rupert: Really?
Ms. Terasaki: First the doctor will finish the examination,

場面：前章の対話の続き。ルパート氏は口腔清掃を終えるために再来院している。

寺崎さん：この間のアポイントの後、歯ぐきはどんな調子でしたか？

ルパート氏：ずいぶん調子が良くなりましたよ。りんごを食べると、いつも出血しましたけれど、今は、もう、出血がありません。

寺崎：それは良かったですね。他に痛いところはありますか？

ルパート氏：奥の右下が少し冷たいものに過敏なんです。

寺崎：それは、クリーニングするとよく起こることです。過敏なのは2～3週間すればなくなるはずです。

ルパート氏：私の歯ぐきの病気は、今日でもうなおるのですか？

寺崎：いいえ、これは長い時間かかりますし、患者さんの努力が必要です。磨き方、フロスの仕方、それに毎日の歯のケアの仕方を覚えていただかなければなりません。

ルパート氏：でも、今日クリーニングを終えてくださるんでしょう？

寺崎：私の方は終りですが、歯医者がポケットのディープ・クリーニングをしなければなりません。これは、もっと深いポケットから歯石を取り除くことをしますし、歯ぐきの手術をする必要があるかもしれません。

ルパート氏：本当ですか？

寺崎：まず先生が診察を終えて、歯ぐきがどの程度なおっ

evaluate how the gums are healing, and make a detailed treatment plan.

Mr. Rupert: I might be here a long time.

Ms. Terasaki: That's right. The treatment may take several visits.

　　　　　　　ているか見きわめて、それから詳しい治療計画を立
　　　　　　　てます。
ルパート氏：ここに長期間来ることになるかもしれませんね。
　　寺崎：そのとおりです。治療は数回来院していただくこと
　　　　　　　になるかもしれません。

Exercises

I. Substitute the following expressions in the example sentence.

Remember to ask him if he <u>feels better</u>.
⟨feels O.K.⟩
Remember to ask him if he <u>feels O.K.</u>

1. feels bad
2. is uncomfortable
3. knows how to find the office
4. brushes regularly
5. understands
6. knows about gum disease
7. has a good toothbrush
8. has any health problems
9. wants a cleaning
10. will return next week
11. wants a new toothbrush
12. found a good dentist

II. Substitute the following expressions in the example sentence.

It is important to know if <u>there are any problems</u>.
⟨the patient is comfortable⟩
It is important to know if <u>the patient is comfortable</u>.

練習問題

Ⅰ．例文の下線部を以下の語句に置き換えなさい。

彼に、前より気分がいいかどうか、忘れずに尋ねなさい。
〈気分がいい〉
彼に、気分がいいかどうか、忘れずに尋ねなさい。

1. 気分が悪い
2. 快適でない
3. 診療所へ来る方法を知っている
4. 規則正しく磨く
5. わかる
6. 歯ぐきの病気について知っている
7. 良い歯ブラシを持っている
8. 何か健康に問題がある
9. クリーニングしてほしい
10. 来週また来る
11. 新しい歯ブラシがほしい
12. 良い歯医者をみつけた

Ⅱ．例文の下線部を以下の語句に置き換えなさい。

問題があるかどうか知ることが大切である。
〈患者が快適である〉
患者が快適であるかどうか知ることが大切である。

1. the patient is happy with the treatment
2. the treatment is a success
3. the patient has a good toothbrush
4. the patient will keep his appointment
5. there is a problem with payment
6. there is a large cavity
7. gum disease is present
8. he will take care of his teeth
9. the situation is hopeless
10. the hygienist is good
11. the patient has a history of diabetes
12. the patient has a history of broken appointments

Ⅲ. Substitute the following expressions in the example sentence.

My <u>gums</u> used to <u>bleed</u>.
⟨breath/smell bad⟩
My <u>breath</u> used to <u>smell bad</u>.

1. teeth/ache
2. teeth/be black
3. hygienist/complain to me
4. dentist/hurt me
5. teeth/bother me
6. mouth/smell
7. denture/fit badly
8. oral hygiene/be poor

1. 患者が治療に満足している
2. 治療がうまくいく
3. 患者が良い歯ブラシを持っている
4. 患者がアポイントを守る
5. 支払いに関して問題がある
6. 大きいむし歯がある
7. 歯ぐきの病気がある
8. 彼が歯のケアをする
9. 状況がどうしようもない
10. 歯科衛生士が良い
11. 患者が糖尿病になったことがある
12. 患者がアポイントを破ったことがある

Ⅲ．例文の下線部を以下の語句に置き換えなさい。

以前は、私の歯ぐきは出血したものだ。
〈息／くさい臭いがする〉
以前は、私の息はくさい臭いがしたものだ。

1. 歯／痛む
2. 歯／黒い
3. 歯科衛生士／私に文句を言う
4. 歯医者／私に痛いことをする
5. 歯／私を悩ませる
6. 口／臭いがする
7. 義歯／フィットが悪い
8. 口腔衛生／悪い

9. attitude/be poor
10. dentist/complain to me
11. gums/hurt every day
12. teeth/be mobile

Ⅳ. Substitute the following expressions in the example sentence.

It may be necessary to <u>do gum surgery</u>.
〈find a good dentist〉
It may be necessary to <u>find a good dentist</u>.

1. find a good pedodontist
2. see a specialist
3. extract the wisdom tooth
4. get a second opinion
5. have a dentist look at the situation
6. repeat the oral hygiene instructions
7. have another cleaning appointment
8. make a new denture
9. take X-rays
10. do a gingivectomy
11. perform a flap operation
12. re-evaluate the periodontal condition

9. 態度／悪い
10. 歯医者／私に文句を言う
11. 歯ぐき／毎日痛む
12. 歯／動く

Ⅳ．例文の下線部を以下の語句に置き換えなさい。

歯ぐきの手術をする必要があるかもしれません。
〈良い歯医者をみつける〉
良い歯医者をみつける必要があるかもしれません。

1. 良い小児歯科医をみつける
2. 専門医に会う
3. 親知らずを抜く
4. 他の（医者の）意見を聞く
5. 歯医者にその状態を見てもらう
6. 口腔衛生指導を繰り返す
7. もう1回、クリーニングのためアポイントをとる
8. 新しい義歯を作る
9. エックス線写真を撮る
10. 歯肉切除術をする
11. 歯肉剥離掻爬術をする
12. 歯周状態を再評価する

V. Substitute the following expressions in the example sentence.

Can you explain what you will do?
⟨what the dentist will do⟩
Can you explain what the dentist will do?

1. how to brush properly
2. why brushing is necessary
3. how to floss
4. how to take care of your teeth
5. what is plaque
6. how to destroy plaque
7. how to clean the teeth
8. how to remove calculus
9. how to prepare the medicine
10. what will be necessary
11. what is gum disease
12. how to clean teeth

Ⅴ．例文の下線部を以下の語句に置き換えなさい。

あなたが何をするのか説明していただけますか？
〈歯医者が何をするのか〉
歯医者が何をするのか説明していただけますか？

1. 正しい磨き方を
2. なぜブラッシングが必要か
3. どのようにしてフロスするか
4. どのようにしてあなたの歯のケアをするか
5. プラークとは何か
6. どのようにしてプラークを壊すか
7. どのようにしてその歯をきれいにするか
8. どのようにして歯石を除去するか
9. どのようにして薬を調合するか
10. 何が必要か
11. 歯ぐきの病気とは何か
12. どのようにして歯をきれいにするか

Chapter 4

> An explanation of the hygienist's treatment
> Part IV: Completion of the oral prophylaxis

The Gums Are Still Red and Puffed Up.

It is important to give the patient the hand mirror and show him his teeth before and after the cleaning. Most patients are quite surprised at the difference and will often thank the hygienist. Also, point out areas where the gingiva is inflamed and where it is healthy. Show the patient the difference and encourage him to check the gingiva every day.

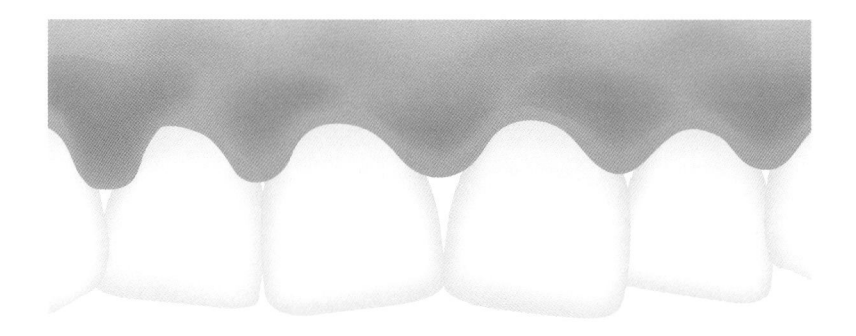

第 4 章

歯科衛生士の処置を患者に説明する
Ⅳ．口腔清掃の仕上げ

歯ぐきがまだ赤くて腫れています

　患者にハンドミラーを渡し、クリーニングの前と後に、歯を見せることが大切である。ほとんどの患者は、その違いにかなり驚くもので、歯科衛生士に感謝することも多い。また、歯肉が炎症を起こしているところと、健康なところを指摘するとよい。患者にその違いを見せて、毎日歯肉をチェックするように勧めなさい。

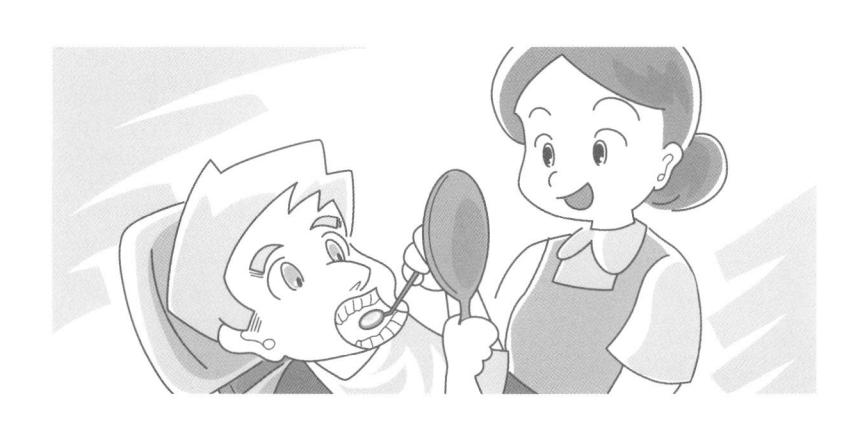

Situation: A continuation of the previous dialogue. Mr. Rupert's cleaning has been finished and he is given the mirror.

Ms. Terasaki: I think we are finished. Would you like to rinse out once more? (She hands the patient a cup of water.)
Mr. Rupert: Yes. Thank you.
Ms. Terasaki: Here is a mirror. Hold it while I place the mouth mirror behind the teeth.
Mr. Rupert: Thank you.
Ms. Terasaki: Can you see how clean the teeth are now?
Mr. Rupert: That looks great!
Ms. Terasaki: There are still some areas where the gums are swollen. Look at the lower front teeth.
Mr. Rupert: Yes. The gums are still red and puffed up.
Ms. Terasaki: This area needs special attention when you brush and floss.
Mr. Rupert: I will be careful to brush well in that area.
Ms. Terasaki: However, the gums around the upper front teeth are quite healthy. Look in the mirror.
Mr. Rupert: Yes. There is a big difference.
Ms. Terasaki: I would like you to check each day in the mirror and watch the lower gums improve.
Mr. Rupert: That's a good idea.

場面：前章の対話の続き。ルパート氏のクリーニングが終ったところで、鏡が渡された。

寺崎さん：これで終ったようですね。もう1度口をゆすがれますか？（水を1杯患者に渡す。）
ルパート氏：ええ。ありがとう。
寺崎：ここに鏡があります。私がミラーを歯の後ろに当てている間、これを持っていてください。
ルパート氏：ありがとう。
寺崎：歯がどんなにきれいになったかご覧になれますか？
ルパート氏：すばらしいですね。
寺崎：まだ、歯ぐきが腫れているところがいくつかあります。下の前歯を見てください。
ルパート氏：ええ。歯ぐきが、まだ赤くて腫れていますね。
寺崎：この部分は、磨いたりフロスする時、特別の注意が必要です。
ルパート氏：そこをよく磨くように気をつけましょう。
寺崎：でも、上の前歯の回りの歯ぐきは健康です。鏡をご覧になってください。
ルパート氏：ええ。ずいぶん違いますね。
寺崎：鏡で毎日チェックして、下の歯ぐきが良くなっていくのを見ていただきたいのです。
ルパート氏：そうしましょう。

Exercises

Ⅰ. Substitute the following expressions in the example sentence.

Encourage the patient to <u>check</u> every day.
⟨brush⟩
Encourage the patient to <u>brush</u> every day.

1. brush his teeth
2. eat good food
3. check his progress in the mirror.
4. avoid sweets
5. use plaque disclosing solution
6. practice brushing
7. use a synthetic bristle toothbrush
8. check his gingival condition
9. take care of his oral health
10. stop smoking
11. floss
12. use the interproximal brush

Ⅱ. Substitute the following expressions in the example sentence.

Mr. Rupert's <u>cleaning</u> has been completed.
⟨treatment⟩
Mr. Rupert's <u>treatment</u> has been completed.

練習問題

Ⅰ．例文の下線部を以下の語句に置き換えなさい。

毎日チェックするように患者に勧めなさい。
〈磨く〉
毎日磨くように患者に勧めなさい。

1. 歯を磨く
2. 良いものを食べる
3. どれぐらいよくなったか鏡でチェックする
4. 甘いものを避ける
5. プラーク染色剤を使う
6. ブラッシングを練習する
7. 合成繊維の歯ブラシを使う
8. 歯肉状態をチェックする
9. 口腔の健康のケアをする
10. たばこをやめる
11. フロスする
12. 歯間ブラシを使う

Ⅱ．例文の下線部を以下の語句に置き換えなさい。

ルパート氏のクリーニングが終ったところ。
〈治療〉
ルパート氏の治療が終ったところ。

1. deep cleaning
2. filling
3. flap operation
4. gum surgery
5. oral prophylaxis
6. oral hygiene instructions (have)
7. initial treatment
8. diagnosis
9. emergency treatment
10. cleaning appointments (have)
11. crown
12. periodontal treatment

Ⅲ. Substitute the following expressions in the example sentence.

This area needs special attention when you brush.
⟨a new restoration⟩
This area needs a new restoration.

1. treatment again
2. extra brushing
3. special attention
4. an interproximal brush
5. flossing
6. more polishing
7. gum surgery
8. root planing and curettage

1. ディープ・クリーニング
2. 充填
3. 歯肉剥離掻爬術
4. 歯ぐきの手術
5. 口腔清掃
6. 口腔衛生指導
7. 初期治療
8. 診断
9. 救急治療
10. クリーニングのアポイント
11. クラウン
12. 歯周病の治療

Ⅲ. 例文の下線部を以下の語句に置き換えなさい。

この部分は、<u>磨く時、特別に注意</u>が必要です。
〈新しい修復〉
この部分は、<u>新しい修復</u>が必要です。

1. もう一度治療すること
2. 余分にブラッシングすること
3. 特別な注意
4. 歯間ブラシ
5. フロッシング
6. 研磨がもっと
7. 歯ぐきの手術
8. ルートプレーニングと掻爬

9. root canal therapy
10. immediate treatment
11. more cleaning
12. to be checked again

Ⅳ. Substitute the following expressions in the example sentence.

I would like you to check every day.
〈brush every day〉
I would like you to brush every day.

1. visit the dentist every six months
2. floss every day
3. stop eating candy
4. make an appointment
5. reschedule the appointment
6. demonstrate your brushing technique
7. find a new toothbrush
8. visit my office
9. brush and floss daily
10. stop talking while I am cleaning your teeth
11. eat good food every day
12. stop drinking cola

9. 根管治療
10. すぐに治療すること
11. クリーニングがもっと
12. もう一度チェックすること

Ⅳ. 例文の下線部を以下の語句に置き換えなさい。

毎日チェックしていただきたいと思います。
〈毎日磨く〉
毎日磨いていただきたいと思います。

1. 6ヵ月ごとに歯医者を訪れる
2. 毎日フロスする
3. キャンディを食べるのをやめる
4. アポイントを取る
5. アポイントし直す
6. ブラッシング・テクニックを見せる
7. 新しい歯ブラシを捜す
8. 私の診療所に来る
9. 毎日歯を磨いてフロスする
10. 私が歯をクリーニングしている間、しゃべるのをやめる
11. 毎日良いものを食べる
12. コーラを飲むのをやめる

V. Substitute the following expressions in the example sentence.

Do you have any questions about how to brush?
〈find the office〉
Do you have any questions about how to find the office?

1. clean your teeth
2. help your child clean his teeth
3. stop bad breath
4. prevent future tooth decay
5. prevent future problems
6. prevent gum disease
7. select a good toothbrush
8. eat properly
9. avoid costly dental treatment
10. take care of your teeth
11. make an appointment
12. decrease tooth decay

Ⅴ．例文の下線部を以下の語句に置き換えなさい。

<u>歯磨き</u>の方法について、何かご質問はありますか？
（診療所をみつける）
<u>診療所をみつける</u>方法について、何かご質問はありますか？

1. 歯をきれいにする
2. あなたの子どもさんが歯をきれいにするのを手伝う
3. 口臭を止める
4. これからのむし歯を防ぐ
5. これからの問題を防ぐ
6. 歯ぐきの病気を防ぐ
7. よい歯ブラシを選ぶ
8. 正しく食べる
9. 高い歯科治療を避ける
10. 歯のケアをする
11. アポイントを取る
12. むし歯を減らす

Chapter 5

A small child's first visit with the hygienist
Part I: An explanation of what will be done

You're Not So Bad After All.

    Sometimes small children are quite frightened during their first few visits to the dentist's office. Their fear may be caused by bad experiences their friends have told them about or by fear of the unknown. It is important to tell little children what you will do. Be sure to use words they can understand.

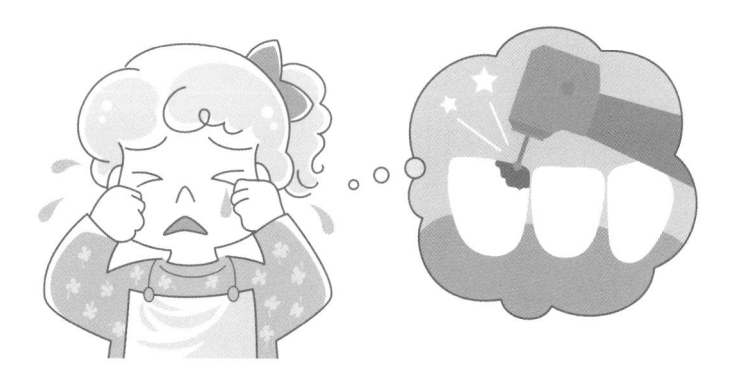

第 5 章

小さな子どもが初めて歯科衛生士と接する時
Ⅰ．何をするか説明する

お姉さんも
そんなに悪くないね

　小さな子どもたちは、歯科医院を訪れるとき初めのうちは恐怖感を持っていることが多い。その恐怖は、友達のひどい経験を聞かされたことから生れたものかもしれないし、また、未知のものに対する恐怖かもしれない。小さな子どもたちには、あなたが何をしようとしているのか説明することが大切である。そして、子どもにも理解できる言葉を使うようにしなければならない。

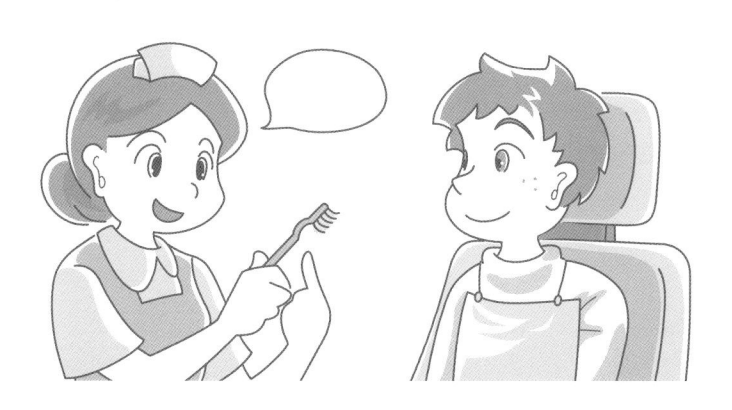

Situation: Bobby Morris, who is four years old, came to the clinic one week ago for a dental examination. Although he had no cavities, there was extensive plaque on his teeth and a special appointment was scheduled for brushing instructions, cleaning, and a topical fluoride treatment. He is a bit nervous and does not seem to understand what the hygienist will do.

Ms. Kano (dental hygienist): Good afternoon Bobby. How are you today?

Bobby: Who are you?

Ms. Kano: My name is Miss Kano. I am going to help you clean your teeth today and teach you how to clean them yourself at home.

Bobby: I brushed them last week. Isn't that enough?

Ms. Kano: No. You should brush three times every day. Also, today I am going to put some fluoride on the teeth to make them strong.

Bobby: Are you going to drill on my teeth, too?

Ms. Kano: No. I don't have any drills. All I will do is clean your teeth and make them strong.

Bobby: Are you sure you won't hurt me?

Ms. Kano: Of course I won't hurt you. If I do anything that you don't like, tell me and I will stop.

Bobby: O.K., I will. But how long will this take?

Ms. Kano: It will take about twenty-five minutes. We should hurry because I have to be home by 5:30 to watch

場面：4歳のボビー・モリスは、1週間前に、歯科検診のために来院した。むし歯はなかったけれど、歯にプラークがたくさんついていたので、歯磨き指導、クリーニング、フッ素の歯面塗布のために、特別のアポイントが取られた。ボビーは、少し神経質になっており、歯科衛生士がこれから何をするのかわかっていない様子である。

加納さん（歯科衛生士）：こんにちは、ボビー。元気？

ボビー：お姉さん、誰？
　加納：私の名前は加納っていいます。今日は、ボビーの歯をきれいにするのを手伝ってあげましょうね。それから、おうちでどうしたらきれいに歯が磨けるか教えてあげましょう。
ボビー：先週磨いたけど、それじゃあだめなの？
　加納：毎日3回磨かなくちゃいけないのよ。それに今日は、歯が強くなるようにフッ素を塗ってあげましょう。

ボビー：歯に穴を開けるの？
　加納：いいえ。私はドリルは持っていないの。私がするのは、あなたの歯をきれいにして強くすることだけよ。
ボビー：本当に痛いことはしないの？
　加納：もちろんしないわ。もし、私が嫌なことをしたら、言ってちょうだい。すぐにやめるから。
ボビー：わかった。そうするよ。だけど、どのくらい時間がかかるの？
　加納：大体25分ぐらいね。ちょっと急がなくちゃいけないわ。ミッキーマウスをテレビで見るために5時30分までに家に

Mickey Mouse on television.
Bobby: You don't watch Mickey Mouse, do you?
Ms. Kano: Sure I do. I watch him every day.
Bobby: You're not so bad after all.

　　　　帰りたいの。
ボビー：お姉さんはミッキーマウスなんて見ないでしょう？
　加納：もちろん見てるわ。毎日見てるのよ。
ボビー：お姉さんもそんなに悪くないね。

Exercises

Ⅰ. Substitute the following expressions in the example sentence.

It is important to tell little children <u>what you will do</u>.

〈who you are〉
It is important to tell little children <u>who you are</u>.

1. your name
2. what sugar bugs* are
3. how to use a toothbrush
4. how to brush
5. where to find sugar bugs
6. about teeth
7. how many teeth they have
8. that teeth are important
9. how to clean their teeth
10. that they have beautiful teeth
11. not to eat sweets
12. to avoid junk food**

* "Sugar bugs" is a word you can use to describe plaque to children. It should only be used when talking with children.
** "Junk food" is a word often used to describe food which is low in nutrition and contains much sugar, fat, or salt. Examples of "junk food" include soft drinks, potato chips, candy, and hot dogs.

練習問題

Ⅰ．例文の下線部を以下の語句に置き換えなさい。

小さな子どもたちには、あなたが何をしようとしているのか教えてあげることが大切である。
〈あなたが誰であるか〉
小さな子どもたちには、あなたが誰であるか教えてあげることが大切である。

1. あなたの名前を
2. 砂糖の虫＊とは何か
3. 歯ブラシの使い方を
4. 磨き方を
5. 砂糖の虫はどこにいるか
6. 歯について
7. 歯が何本あるか
8. 歯は大切だと
9. 歯をきれいにする方法を
10. きれいな歯をしていると
11. 甘いものを食べないように
12. ジャンクフード＊＊を避けるように

＊「砂糖の虫」とは子どもにプラークを説明する言葉で、子どもと話す時だけ使うのが良い。
＊＊「ジャンクフード」とは、栄養価が低く、砂糖、脂肪、塩分などを多く含む食品をいう言葉である。ジャンクフードには、清涼飲料水、ポテトチップス、キャンディ、ホットドッグなどがある。

II. Substitute the following expressions in the example sentence.

A special appointment was scheduled for brushing instructions.
⟨flossing instructions⟩
A special appointment was scheduled for flossing instructions.

1. instructions
2. a fluoride treatment
3. oral hygiene instructions
4. instructions for the parents
5. amalgam restorations
6. his parents
7. cleaning his teeth
8. a complete examination
9. X-rays
10. some reason
11. my treatment
12. periodontal surgery

III. Substitute the following expressions in the example sentence.

I'm going to help you clean your teeth.
⟨hunt for sugar bugs⟩
I'm going to help you hunt for sugar bugs.

1. hunt for plaque

Ⅱ．例文の下線部を以下の語句に置き換えなさい。

<u>歯磨き指導</u>のために、特別なアポイントが取られた。
〈フロスの指導〉
<u>フロスの指導</u>のために、特別なアポイントが取られた。

1. 指導
2. フッ素の応用
3. 口腔衛生指導
4. 親のための指導
5. アマルガム修復
6. 彼の両親
7. 歯のクリーニング
8. 完全な診査
9. エックス線写真
10. 何らかの理由
11. 私の治療
12. 歯周外科

Ⅲ．例文の下線部を以下の語句に置き換えなさい。

<u>歯をきれいにする</u>のを手伝ってあげましょう。
〈砂糖の虫をつかまえる〉
<u>砂糖の虫をつかまえる</u>のを手伝ってあげましょう。

1. プラークをみつける

2. floss your teeth

3. take care of your oral health

4. prevent decay

5. find sugar bugs

6. get rid of those sugar bugs

7. prevent gum disease

8. use the toothbrush

9. use the floss

10. clean your mouth

11. clean off the plaque disclosing solution

12. prevent new decay

Ⅳ. Substitute the following expressions in the example sentence

I have to be home by 5:30 to watch Mickey Mouse.

〈brush my teeth〉

I have to be home by 5:30 to brush my teeth.

1. practice brushing my teeth
2. buy a new toothbrush before the store closes
3. help my sister floss her teeth
4. clean my teeth
5. floss my teeth
6. take care of my teeth
7. show my mother my clean teeth
8. get ready for my dental appointment

2. 歯をフロスする
3. 口腔の健康のケアをする
4. むし歯を防ぐ
5. 砂糖の虫を探す
6. 砂糖の虫を追い払う
7. 歯ぐきの病気を防ぐ
8. 歯ブラシを使う
9. フロスを使う
10. 口をきれいにする
11. プラーク染色剤をきれいに取る
12. 新しいむし歯を防ぐ

Ⅳ．例文の下線部を以下の語句に置き換えなさい。

<u>ミッキーマウスを見る</u>ために、5時30分までに家に帰らなければなりません。
〈歯を磨く〉
<u>歯を磨く</u>ために、5時30分までに家に帰らなければなりません。

1. ブラッシングを練習する
2. お店が閉店する前に新しい歯ブラシを買う
3. 姉（妹）がフロスするのを手伝う
4. 歯をきれいにする
5. 歯をフロスする
6. 歯のケアをする
7. 母にきれいな歯を見せる
8. 歯医者に行くため用意する

9. help my brother brush his teeth
10. practice flossing my teeth
11. clean my teeth before the dental appointment
12. get dressed for my dental appointment

Ⅴ. Substitute the following expressions in the example dialogue.

- You don't <u>watch Mickey Mouse</u>, do you?
- Sure I do. I <u>watch him</u> every day.
- You're not so bad after all.

⟨brush your teeth/brush them⟩

- You don't <u>brush your teeth</u>, do you?
- Sure I do. I <u>brush them</u> every day.
- You're not so bad after all.

1. brush your child's teeth/brush them
2. clean your teeth/clean them
3. floss your teeth/floss them
4. floss/floss
5. avoid sweets/avoid them
6. avoid junk foods/avoid them
7. take care of your teeth/take care of them
8. use a synthetic bristle toothbrush/use it
9. use a soft bristle toothbrush/use it
10. use plaque disclosing solution/use it
11. avoid hard candies/avoid them
12. clean children's teeth/clean them

9. 兄（弟）が歯を磨くのを手伝う
10. フロッシングを練習する
11. 歯医者さんとのアポイントの前に歯をきれいにする
12. 歯医者に行くため服を着る

Ⅴ．例にあげた対話の下線部を以下の語句に置き換えなさい。

－<u>ミッキーマウスなんて見ない</u>でしょう？
－もちろん見ているわ。毎日<u>見</u>ているのよ。
－あなたもそんなに悪くないね。
〈歯を磨く〉
－<u>歯なんて磨かない</u>でしょう？
－もちろん磨くわ。毎日<u>磨</u>いているのよ。
－あなたもそんなに悪くないね。

1. 子どもの歯を磨く
2. 歯をきれいにする
3. 歯をフロスする
4. フロスする
5. 甘いものを避ける
6. ジャンクフードを避ける
7. 歯のケアをする
8. 合成繊維の毛の歯ブラシを使う
9. 柔らかい毛の歯ブラシを使う
10. プラーク染色剤を使う
11. 固いキャンディを避ける
12. 子どもたちの歯をきれいにする

Chapter 6

A small child's first visit with the hygienist
Part II: An explanation of the instruments and equipment

Sometimes Sugar Bugs Hide Between the Teeth.

Small children may be frightened during their first visit with the hygienist simply because they are not familiar with the new place and new instruments. It is important to show them each of the instruments you will use and explain how they will be used. The air syringe is called Mr. Wind; the water syringe, Mr. Rain.

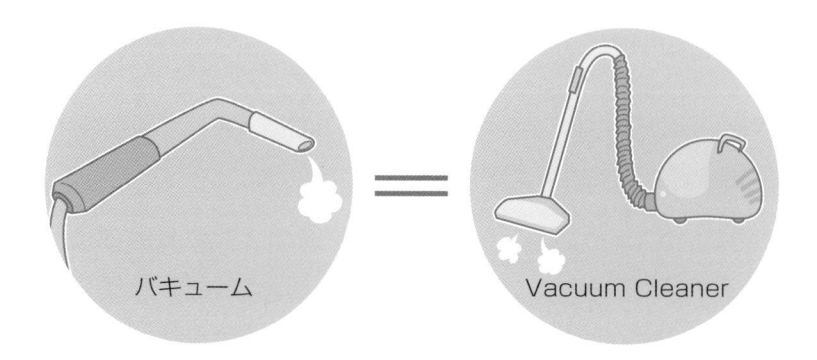

バキューム = Vacuum Cleaner

第 6 章

小さな子どもが初めて歯科衛生士と接する時
Ⅱ．器具や設備の説明

時々、砂糖の虫は歯と歯の間に隠れているの

　小さな子どもが初めて歯科衛生士と接する時、初めの頃は、新しい場所や、新しい器具を見慣れていないというだけの理由で、怖がるかもしれない。あなたが使う器具をひとつひとつ見せて、それがどのように使われるのか説明してあげることが大切である。エアーシリンジはミスター・ウィンド（風さん）、ウォーターシリンジは、ミスター・レイン（雨さん）と呼ばれている。

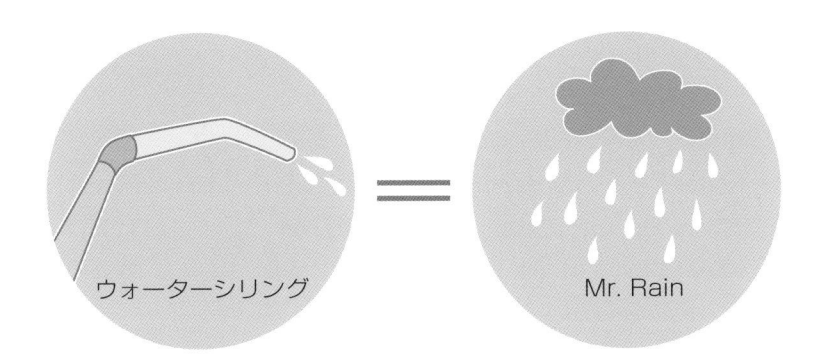

ウォーターシリング ＝ Mr. Rain

Situation: A continuation of the previous dialogue. Bobby is seated in the hygienist's chair.

Bobby: What are all those instruments?
Ms. Kano (dental hygienist): This one is a little mirror for looking at teeth. Do you want to hold it? (She hands the mirror to him.)
Bobby: Yes.
Ms. Kano: And this one is Mr. Wind. (She points the air syringe to her hand and blows the air lightly.) Hold your hand out and I'll show you how it feels.

Bobby: (He holds out his hand.) That feels cool.
Ms. Kano: And this is Mr. Rain. When I push this button, water sprays out. (she sprays a few drops of water into her hand.) I use this for giving your teeth a bath.
Bobby: Wow! My teeth never had a bath!
Ms. Kano: And this is my vacuum cleaner. (She holds the vacuum first against her cheek and then against Bobby's cheek.)
Bobby: That tickles.
Ms. Kano: I use my vacuum cleaner to clean your mouth.

Bobby: Is my mouth dirty?
Ms. Kano: I think there might be a few sugar bugs in there.
Bobby: Then hurry up and get them out.
Ms. Kano: First I'm going to give you a quiz. What is this? (She holds out a toothbrush.)
Bobby: It's a toothbrush.

場面：前の対話の続き。ボビーは歯科衛生士の椅子に座っている。

ボビー：このいろいろな道具は何？
加納さん（歯科衛生士）：これは歯を見るための鏡よ。ちょっと持ってみる？（鏡をボビーに渡す。）

ボビー：うん。
加納：そしてこれはミスター・ウィンドよ。（エアーシリンジを手の方に向けて、軽くエアーを出してみる。）手を出してみてちょうだい。どのように感じるか見せてあげましょう。
ボビー：（手を出す。）冷たいね。
加納：そしてこれがミスター・レインよ。このボタンを押すと、水が吹き出すの。（自分の手に水を2〜3滴スプレーする。）歯をお風呂に入れてあげるためにこれを使うの。
ボビー：わー！僕の歯はお風呂に入ったことないよ。
加納：それから、これが掃除機よ。（バキュームを、最初自分の頬に当て、それからボビーの頬に当てる。）

ボビー：くすぐったいよ。
加納：あなたの歯をきれいにするのに、この掃除機を使いましょう。
ボビー：僕の口は汚い？
加納：そこに砂糖の虫が少しいるかもしれないわ。
ボビー：じゃあ、急いで取って。
加納：最初に、クイズを出しましょう。これは何でしょう。（歯ブラシを出す。）
ボビー：歯ブラシです。

Ms. Kano: That's right. I use this for cleaning your teeth.
    Bobby: How about that string? What is that for?
Ms. Kano: This is floss for cleaning between your teeth. Sometimes sugar bugs hide there.
    Bobby: You have a lot of fun things here.

加納：そのとおり。これを使って歯をきれいにしましょう。
ボビー：その糸は何？　何に使うの？
加納：これは歯と歯の間をそうじするフロスというものよ。
　　　時々、砂糖の虫はそこに隠れているの。
ボビー：ここには、いろんなおもしろいものがあるんだね。

Exercises

Ⅰ. Substitute the following expressions in the example sentence.

Small children may be frightened by <u>the air syringe</u>.
⟨the water syringe⟩
Small children may be frightened by <u>the water syringe</u>.

1. the mirror
2. sugar bugs
3. the hygienist
4. the dentist
5. people wearing white clothes
6. the unknown
7. plaque disclosing solution
8. dental instruments
9. the chair light
10. dental treatment
11. the mouth mirror
12. the sound of the vacuum

Ⅱ. Substitute the following expressions in the example sentence.

I will show you how <u>it feels</u>.
⟨to take care of your teeth⟩
I will show you how <u>to take care of your teeth</u>.

練習問題

Ⅰ．例文の下線部を以下の語句に置き換えなさい。

小さい子どもたちは、エアーシリンジを怖がるかもしれない。
〈ウォーターシリンジ〉
小さい子どもたちは、ウォーターシリンジを怖がるかもしれない。

1. 鏡
2. 砂糖の虫
3. 歯科衛生士
4. 歯医者
5. 白い服を着ている人々
6. 知らないもの
7. プラーク染色剤
8. 歯科医療器具
9. 診療椅子のライト
10. 歯科治療
11. ミラー
12. バキュームの音

Ⅱ．例文の下線部を以下の語句に置き換えなさい。

どのように感じるか見せてあげましょう。
〈歯のケアをする〉
どのように歯のケアをするか見せてあげましょう。

1. to take care of your toothbrush
2. the vacuum cleans your mouth
3. to use plaque disclosing solution
4. to fight decay
5. to prevent gum disease
6. to prevent decay
7. I clean teeth
8. to select a good toothbrush
9. to get rid of all of the plaque
10. to save your teeth
11. my air syringe works
12. to handle children

Ⅲ. Substitute the following expressions in the example dialogue.

- What are you going to do now?
- I'm going to give you a quiz.
⟨teach you how to brush your teeth⟩
- What are you going to do now?
- I'm going to teach you how to brush your teeth.

1. teach you how to brush
2. show you Mr. Rain
3. floss your teeth
4. let you hold the mirror
5. clean your teeth
6. take you to the dentist

1. 歯ブラシのケアをする
2. バキュームがあなたの口をきれいにする
3. プラーク染色剤を使う
4. むし歯と戦う
5. 歯ぐきの病気を防ぐ
6. むし歯を防ぐ
7. 私が歯をきれいにする
8. よい歯ブラシを選ぶ
9. プラークを全部取り除く
10. あなたの歯を助ける
11. 私のエアーシリンジが動く
12. 子どもたちを扱う

Ⅲ．例にあげた対話の下線部を以下の語句に置き換えなさい。

－今から何をするのですか？
－あなたにクイズを出します。
〈あなたに歯の磨き方を教える〉
－今から何をするのですか？
－あなたに歯の磨き方を教えます。

1. あなたに磨き方を教える
2. ミスター・レインを見せる
3. あなたの歯をフロッシングする
4. あなたにミラーを握らせる
5. あなたの歯をきれいにする
6. あなたを歯医者に連れていく

7. help you care for your teeth
8. show you Mr. Wind
9. show you the different instruments
10. put plaque disclosing solution in your mouth
11. help you brush and floss
12. teach you how to floss

Ⅳ. Substitute the following expressions in the example sentence.

Hurry up and <u>get the sugar bugs out of my mouth.</u>
〈brush your teeth〉
Hurry up and <u>brush your teeth.</u>

1. brush
2. clean my teeth
3. buy the toothbrush
4. find the sugar bugs
5. give the brushing instructions
6. learn how to brush
7. teach me how to get rid of sugar bugs
8. clean the child's teeth
9. take care of him
10. get some floss
11. finish the brushing
12. find a good dentist

7. あなたが歯のケアをするのを手伝う
8. ミスター・ウィンドを見せる
9. あなたに違う器具を見せる
10. あなたの口にプラーク染色剤を入れる
11. あなたが歯を磨いてフロッシングするのを手伝う
12. あなたにフロッシングの仕方を教える

Ⅳ．例文の下線部を以下の語句に置き換えなさい。

急いで私の口から砂糖の虫を取って_ください。
〈あなたの歯を磨く〉
急いであなたの歯を磨いて_ください。

1. 磨く
2. 私の歯をきれいにする
3. 歯ブラシを買う
4. 砂糖の虫をみつける
5. 歯ブラシ指導をする
6. 磨き方を覚える
7. 私に砂糖の虫の取り方を教える
8. 子どもの歯をきれいにする
9. 彼の面倒を見る
10. フロスをもらう
11. ブラッシングを終える
12. 良い歯医者をみつける

V. Substitute the following expressions in the example dialogue.

- Is my mouth dirty?
- I think that there might be <u>a few sugar bugs</u> in there.
⟨some plaque⟩
- Is my mouth dirty?
- I think that there might be <u>some plaque</u> in there.

1. too much plaque
2. some candy
3. some food particles
4. a potato chip
5. a cookie
6. sugar
7. a piece of hamburger
8. a little bit of food
9. a piece of ice cream cone
10. a little piece of pizza
11. some noodles
12. a piece of potato chip

Ⅴ．例にあげた対話の下線部を以下の語句に置き換えなさい。

－僕の口は汚い？
－そこに砂糖の虫が少しいるかもしれないわ。
〈プラークがいくらか〉
－僕の口は汚い？
－そこにプラークがいくらかあるかもしれないわ。

1. あまりにもたくさんのプラークが
2. キャンディが少し
3. 食べ物の破片がいくらか
4. ポテトチップスが
5. クッキーが
6. 砂糖が
7. ハンバーガーの小片が
8. 食べ物がほんの少しだけ
9. アイスクリームコーンの小片が
10. ピザの小片が
11. ヌードルがいくらか
12. ポテトチップのかけらが

Chapter 7

A small child's first visit with the hygienist
Part III: Brushing instructions

What Are Sugar Bugs?

The parent should be present during oral hygiene instructions for the child. Children cannot brush effectively until they are at least six years old. Even until the child is twelve years old, it is the parents' responsibility to check how well he is brushing, and to brush and floss his teeth after he has finished. Plaque disclosing solution is a valuable asset in this process.

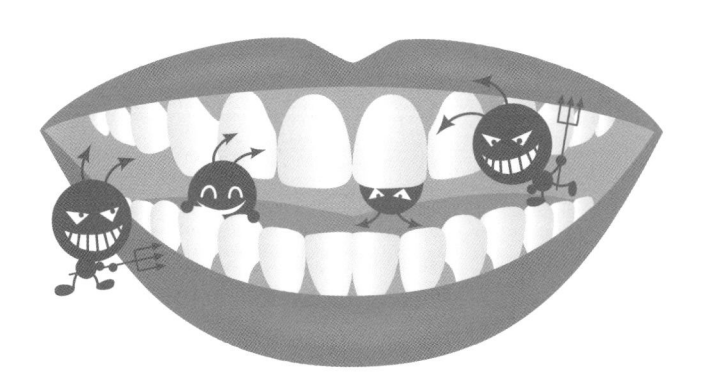

第 7 章

小さな子どもが初めて歯科衛生士と接する時
Ⅲ．歯ブラシ指導

砂糖の虫って何？

　子どもに口腔衛生指導をする間、親もそこにいるべきである。子どもは、少なくとも6歳になるまで、十分に磨けない。子どもが12歳になるまでは、どの程度よく磨いているかチェックし、子どもが磨き終えた後、歯を磨きフロッシングするのは親の責任である。プラーク染色剤は、これをするうえで重要な役割を果たす。

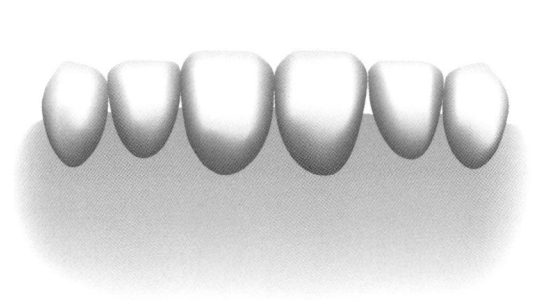

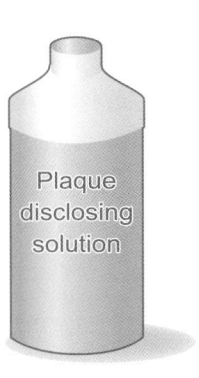

Situation: A continuation of the previous dialogue. The hygienist explains what plaque is, and how to brush and floss. The parent has been brought into the hygienist's room.

Ms. Kano (dental hygienist): Before I clean your teeth, I want to put a little red coloring on them so that we can see the sugar bugs.

Bobby: What are sugar bugs?

Ms. Kano: They are tiny little bugs that live on your teeth. They are so small that you cannot see them. When you eat sweets, the sugar bugs get big and make holes in your teeth.

Bobby: I don't want that.

Ms. Kano: That's why you have to brush your teeth. Brushing cleans the teeth and prevents decay.

Bobby: How can I get rid of sugar bugs if I can't see them?

Ms. Kano: It's easy. First we put this red coloring in your mouth and the sugar bugs all turn red.

Bobby: How long will my mouth be red?

Ms. Kano: The red will go away when you brush your teeth and rinse your mouth.

Bobby: Then let's get on with it. I don't want any sugar bugs in my mouth.

Ms. Kano: O.K., open wide. I'll put in a few drops of coloring. Swish it around in your mouth for thirty seconds. Then rinse your mouth one time with water.

場面：前章の対話の続き。歯科衛生士は、プラークとは何か、また、どのようにして歯を磨きフロスするか説明する。親は歯科衛生士の部屋に呼び入れられた。

加納さん（歯科衛生士）：あなたの歯をきれいにする前に、砂糖の虫が見えるように赤い水を少し歯につけましょう。

ボビー：砂糖の虫って何？
　加納：歯に住んでいる小さな小さな虫よ。とても小さいから見えないの。甘いものを食べると、砂糖の虫が大きくなって歯に穴をあけるの。

ボビー：そんなのいやだ。
　加納：だから歯を磨かなくちゃいけないのよ。磨くと歯がきれいになって、むし歯にもならないわ。
ボビー：でも、もし見えないんだったら、どうやって砂糖の虫をやっつけることができるの？
　加納：それは簡単。まず、この赤い水を歯につけると、砂糖の虫はみんな赤くなるわ。
ボビー：どのくらいのあいだ口が赤くなるの？
　加納：歯を磨いて口をゆすぐと、赤いのはなくなるわ。

ボビー：じゃあ、早くしようよ。砂糖の虫が口の中にいるのはいやだもの。
　加納：そうね。口を大きく開けて2～3滴口の中に染色剤を入れましょう。30秒間口の中でぐちゅぐちゅってしてちょうだい、それから、一度水で口をゆすいでね。

Bobby: O.K. (The hygienist places four drops of plaque disclosing solution in Bobby's mouth. He swishes for thirty seconds and rinses.)

Ms. Kano: Now, look in the mirror.

Bobby: Yucky. Look at all that red stuff on my teeth!

Ms. Kano: Shall I clean off those sugar bugs?

Bobby: Yes! As fast as you can!

Ms. Kano: O.K. Hold this mirror and watch. The first thing we do is to place the brush on the teeth and brush like this in a circle, ten times. Now, look at these three teeth which we brushed.

Bobby: Gee. They're white.

Ms. Kano: That's right. Don't they look nice?

Bobby: Yes. I want all my teeth to look like that.

Ms. Kano: All you have to do is brush just like I showed you.

Bobby: That's easy.

Ms. Kano: And when you finish brushing, be sure to have your mother check to see that all of the sugar bugs are gone and have her brush your teeth again and floss them.

Bobby: O.K.

ボビー：オーケー（歯科衛生士はボビーの口に、プラーク染色剤を4滴入れる。ボビーは30秒間ぐちゅぐちゅしてから、口をゆすぐ。）

加納：さあ、鏡を見て。

ボビー：気持ち悪い。歯についてる赤いのを見てよ。

加納：砂糖の虫を取ってきれいにしてあげましょうか？

ボビー：うん。できるだけ早くね。

加納：わかりました。この鏡を持って見ていてちょうだい。初めにするのは、ブラシを歯の上に当てて、10回このようにぐるぐると丸く磨くこと。ほら、今磨いた3本の歯を見てご覧なさい。

ボビー：わあ。白いね。

加納：そのとおり。すてきじゃない？

ボビー：そうだね。僕の歯が全部こんなだといいな。

加納：私がして見せたみたいに磨きさえすればいいの。

ボビー：簡単だね。

加納：そして磨き終えたら、必ず、お母さんに砂糖の虫がいなくなっているかどうかチェックしてもらって、歯をもう一度磨いてフロスもしてもらってね。

ボビー：オーケー。

Exercises

Ⅰ. Substitute the following expressions in the example sentence.

It is the parents' responsibility to brush the child's teeth.
⟨take care of the child⟩
It is the parents' responsibility to take care of the child.

1. take the child to the dentist
2. brush their own teeth to set a good example
3. make the appointment
4. help the child
5. help the child with disclosing solution
6. floss the child's teeth
7. buy the toothpaste
8. buy the toothbrush
9. buy the dental floss
10. contact the dentist
11. care for their child's teeth
12. care for their children's teeth

Ⅱ. Substitute the following expressions in the example sentence.

I don't want any sugar bugs in my mouth.
⟨any plaque⟩
I don't want any plaque in my mouth.

練習問題

Ⅰ．例文の下線部を以下の語句に置き換えなさい。

<u>子どもの歯を磨く</u>のは、親の責任である。
〈子どもの世話をする〉
<u>子どもの世話をする</u>のは、親の責任である。

1. 子どもを歯医者に連れていく
2. 自分自身の歯を磨いてよいお手本を見せる
3. アポイントを取る
4. 子どもを助ける
5. 子どもが染め出しをするのを手伝う
6. 子どもの歯をフロッシングする
7. 歯磨きを買う
8. 歯ブラシを買う
9. デンタルフロスを買う
10. 歯医者に連絡する
11. 子どもの歯のケアをする
12. 子どもたちの歯のケアをする

Ⅱ．例文の下線部を以下の語句に置き換えなさい。

<u>砂糖の虫</u>が口の中にあるのはいやだ。
〈プラーク〉
<u>プラーク</u>が口の中にあるのはいやだ。

1. a mirror
2. cavities
3. a toothbrush
4. silver fillings
5. amalgam fillings
6. any gold
7. any candy
8. sweets
9. your fingers
10. a bad taste
11. any more fillings
12. any more cavities

Ⅲ. Substitute the following expressions in the example dialogue.

− Shall I clean those sugar bugs off your teeth?
− Yes! As fast as you can!
⟨your mouth⟩
− Shall I clean your mouth?
− Yes! As fast as you can!

1. your molars
2. your teeth
3. the red stain
4. the front teeth
5. the back teeth
6. the stain off your teeth

1. 鏡
2. むし歯
3. 歯ブラシ
4. 銀の充填物
5. アマルガムの充填物
6. 金
7. キャンディ
8. 甘いもの
9. あなたの指
10. 悪い味
11. これ以上たくさんの充填物
12. これ以上たくさんのむし歯

Ⅲ．例にあげた対話の下線部を以下の語句に置き換えなさい。

－<u>砂糖の虫を取って歯を</u>きれいにしてあげましょうか？
－うん。できるだけ早くね。
〈あなたの口〉
－<u>あなたの口を</u>きれいにしてあげましょうか？
－うん。できるだけ早くね。

1. あなたの臼歯
2. あなたの歯
3. 赤い染み
4. 前歯
5. 奥歯
6. ステインをとった歯

7. all your teeth

8. the patient's teeth

9. the child's teeth

10. the child's face

11. the crown

12. the porcelain tooth

Ⅳ. Substitute the following expressions in the example dialogue.

− Why do I have to brush my teeth?
− Brushing cleans the teeth and prevents <u>decay</u>.
⟨tooth decay⟩
− Why do I have to brush my teeth?
− Brushing cleans the teeth and prevents <u>tooth decay</u>.

1. carious lesions

2. holes in your teeth

3. problems

4. bad breath

5. cavities

6. cavities and bad breath

7. ugly teeth

8. early loss of teeth

9. sugar bugs

10. dirty teeth

11. visits to the dentist's office

12. the need for fillings

7. 全部の歯
  8. 患者の歯
  9. 子どもの歯
 10. 子どもの顔
 11. クラウン
 12. 陶歯

Ⅳ．例にあげた対話の下線部を以下の語句に置き換えなさい。

－なぜ歯を磨かなければいけないんですか？
－磨くと歯がきれいになって、むし歯になりません。
〈むし歯〉
－なぜ歯を磨かなければいけないんですか？
－磨くと歯がきれいになって、むし歯になりません。

  1. う蝕
  2. 歯に穴があくこと
  3. いろいろな問題
  4. 口臭
  5. むし歯
  6. むし歯と口臭
  7. 醜い歯
  8. 歯を早く失ってしまうこと
  9. 砂糖の虫（を防ぎます）
 10. きたない歯
 11. 歯医者の診療所に行く（必要がなくなる）
 12. 充填物が必要

Ⅴ. Substitute the following expressions in the example dialogue.

- Have you finished brushing your teeth?
- No, not yet.

⟨flossing⟩

- Have you finished flossing?
- No, not yet.

1. cleaning the teeth
2. flossing your teeth
3. cleaning the child's teeth
4. filling the teeth
5. cleaning the molars
6. instructing the patient
7. using the plaque disclosing solution
8. using the floss
9. rinsing your mouth
10. treating the patient
11. the brushing instructions
12. removing the calculus

Ⅴ．例にあげた対話の下線部を以下の語句に置き換えなさい。

－歯を磨き終えましたか？
－いいえ。まだです。
〈フロッシングする〉
－フロッシングし終えましたか？
－いいえ。まだです。

1. 歯をきれいにする
2. 歯をフロッシングする
3. 子どもの歯をきれいにする
4. 歯をつめる
5. 臼歯をきれいにする
6. 患者に指示を与える
7. プラーク染色剤を使う
8. フロスを使う
9. 口をゆすぐ
10. 患者を治療する
11. ブラッシング指導
12. 歯石を除去する

Chapter 8

A small child's first visit with the hygienist
Part IV: Flossing instructions

Those Sugar Bugs Were Hiding Everywhere.

As with brushing, the parent should be in the room while flossing is explained. Children less than twelve years old usually cannot floss their own teeth properly. It is the parents' responsibility to floss the child's teeth every day.

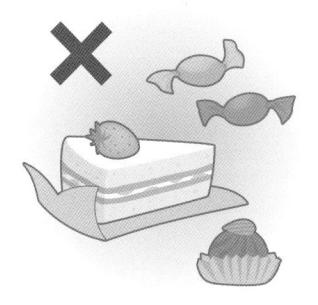

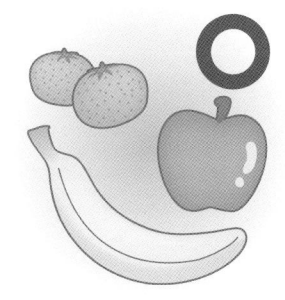

第 8 章

小さな子どもが初めて歯科衛生士と接する時
Ⅳ．フロッシング指導

その砂糖の虫はいろんなところに隠れていたんだね

　ブラッシング指導と同様に、フロスの説明をするときも親が同席するべきである。12歳以下の子どもたちは、普通、自分の歯をきちんとフロスすることができない。子どもの歯を毎日フロスするのは親の責任である。

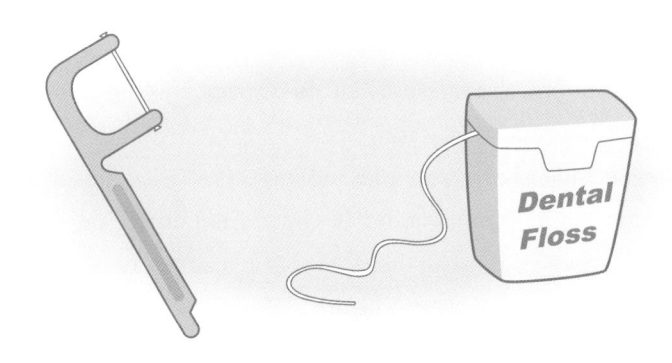

Situation: A continuation of the previous dialogue. Bobby is being taught about flossing.

Ms. Kano: Now, I am going to use this floss to clean between the teeth.
Bobby: Why do you want to do that?
Ms. Kano: Some sugar bugs are hiding there.
Bobby: Well, let's get them out.
Ms. Kano: First I put the floss between the teeth.
Bobby: That tickles.
Ms. Kano: Then I move the floss up and down to get out the sugar bugs. Look at the floss. It's red.

Bobby: Those sugar bugs were hiding everywhere.
Ms. Kano: But we got them all out.
Bobby: Now can I eat some candy?
Ms. Kano: How about eating something good for your teeth like an apple?
Bobby: My father said the same thing.
Ms. Kano: (speaking to Mr. Morris) It is the parents' responsibility to floss Bobby's teeth every day.
Mr. Morris: Shouldn't he do that?
Ms. Kano: Bobby is too young to do a proper job of flossing by himself.
Mr. Morris: That seems like a lot of work.
Ms. Kano: But it is important. If you do not make an effort to help him clean his teeth, you cannot expect him to value good dental health.
Mr. Morris: I suppose that is right.

場面：前章の対話の続き。ボビーはフロスについて教えてもらっている。

加納さん：さあ、歯と歯の間をこのフロスできれいにしてあげましょう。
ボビー：どうしてそんなことしたいの？
加納：砂糖の虫の中には、そこに隠れているのもいるからよ。
ボビー：じゃあ、追い出しちゃおうよ。
加納：まず、歯の間にフロスを入れましょう。
ボビー：くすぐったいよ。
加納：それから、砂糖の虫を追い出すために、フロスを上げたり下げたりします。フロスを見てください。赤いでしょう。
ボビー：その砂糖の虫はいろんなところに隠れていたんだね。
加納：でも、全部追い出してしまったわ。
ボビー：もうキャンディ食べてもいい？
加納：りんごみたいに何か歯によい物を食べたらどうかしら？
ボビー：僕のお父さんも同じこと言ったよ。
加納：（モリス氏に話しかけて）ボビーの歯を毎日フロスするのは親の責任です。
モリス氏：ボビーがするべきじゃありませんか？
加納：ボビーは、自分できちんとフロスするにはまだ小さすぎるのです。
モリス氏：なかなか手間がかかりますね。
加納：でも大切です。もしあなたが努力してボビーが歯をきれいにするのを手伝わなかったら、彼が歯の健康を大切にするのは望めないでしょう。
モリス氏：そうでしょうね。

Exercises

Ⅰ. Substitute the following expressions in the example sentence.

It is the hygienist's job to <u>floss</u> the child's teeth.
⟨brush⟩
It is the hygienist's job to <u>brush</u> the child's teeth.

1. brush and floss
2. take care of
3. clean
4. use floss on
5. put plaque disclosing solution on
6. thoroughly brush
7. get sugar bugs off
8. remove plaque from
9. remove stain from
10. remove food debris from
11. remove the plaque disclosing solution from
12. thoroughly clean

Ⅱ. Substitute the following expressions in the example dialogue.

－Now can I eat some candy?
－How about eating something good for your teeth like <u>an apple</u>?
⟨a pear⟩
－Now can I eat some candy?

練習問題

Ⅰ．例文の下線部を以下の語句に置き換えなさい。

子どもの歯を<u>フロッシングする</u>のは、歯科衛生士の仕事です。
〈磨く〉
子どもの歯を<u>磨く</u>のは、歯科衛生士の仕事です。

1. 磨いてフロッシングする
2. ケアする
3. きれいにする
4. （歯に）フロスを使う
5. （歯に）プラーク染色剤をつける
6. 完全に磨く
7. （歯から）砂糖の虫を取る
8. （歯から）プラークを除去する
9. （歯から）ステインを除去する
10. （歯から）食べかすを除去する
11. （歯から）プラーク染色剤を除去する
12. 完全にきれいにする

Ⅱ．例にあげた対話の下線部を以下の語句に置き換えなさい。

－もうキャンディ食べてもいい？
－<u>りんご</u>みたいに何か歯によい物を食べたらどうかしら？
〈なし〉
－もうキャンディ食べてもいい？

− How about eating something good for your teeth like a pear?

1. a grape
2. a peach
3. some celery
4. a carrot
5. an orange
6. some cheese
7. some vegetables
8. some fruit
9. a carrot stick
10. some apples
11. a tomato
12. some lettuce

Ⅲ. Substitute the following expressions in the example sentence.

Why do you want to do that?
⟨get cavities⟩
Why do you want to get cavities?

1. get holes in your teeth
2. go to the dentist
3. floss my teeth
4. get rid of sugar bugs
5. brush my teeth
6. eat sweets

－なしみたいに何か歯によい物を食べたらどうかしら？

1. ぶどう
2. もも
3. セロリ
4. にんじん
5. オレンジ
6. チーズ
7. 野菜
8. フルーツ
9. にんじんのスティック
10. りんごをいくつか
11. トマト
12. レタス

Ⅲ．例文の下線部を以下の語句に置き換えなさい。

どうしてそんなことしたいの？
〈むし歯になる〉
どうしてむし歯になりたいの？

1. 歯に穴をあける
2. 歯医者に行く
3. 私の歯をフロッシングする
4. 砂糖の虫を追い出す
5. 私の歯を磨く
6. 甘いものを食べる

7. put fluoride on my teeth
8. stop tooth decay
9. prevent gum disease
10. clean my teeth
11. use plaque disclosing tablets
12. put a filling in that tooth

Ⅳ. Substitute the following expressions in the example dialogue.

− What's the hygienist going to do?
− She's going to <u>use this floss to clean your teeth</u>.
⟨remove the plaque⟩
− What's the hygienist going to do?
− She's going to <u>remove the plaque</u>.

1. use this toothbrush
2. clean your teeth
3. brush your teeth
4. do a cleaning
5. rinse your mouth
6. polish your teeth
7. make your teeth whiter
8. use floss
9. put some toothpaste on the toothbrush
10. remove the stain
11. polish the anterior teeth
12. do a fluoride treatment

7. 私の歯にフッ素を塗布する
8. むし歯を止める
9. 歯ぐきの病気を防ぐ
10. 私の歯をきれいにする
11. プラーク染色剤を使う
12. その歯に充填物を入れる

Ⅳ．例にあげた対話の下線部を以下の語句に置き換えなさい。

－歯科衛生士は何をするつもりですか？
－<u>あなたの歯をきれいにするために、このフロスを使う</u>つもりです。
〈プラークを除去する〉
－歯科衛生士は何をするつもりですか？
－<u>プラークを除去する</u>つもりです。

1. この歯ブラシを使う
2. あなたの歯をきれいにする
3. あなたの歯を磨く
4. クリーニングをする
5. あなたの口をゆすぐ
6. あなたの歯を研磨する
7. あなたの歯をもっと白くする
8. フロスを使う
9. 歯ブラシに歯磨きをつける
10. ステインを除去する
11. 前歯を研磨する
12. フッ素を応用する

V. Substitute the following expressions in the example sentence.

My father said the same thing.
⟨to brush my teeth⟩
My father said to brush my teeth.

1. to brush every day
2. to take care of my teeth
3. not to eat junk food
4. not to eat candy
5. to eat nutritious food
6. to use fluoride toothpaste
7. the same thing that you did
8. to brush and floss
9. to eat an apple
10. to floss every day
11. to see a dentist
12. to listen to the dentist

Ⅴ．例文の下線部を以下の語句に置き換えなさい。

私のお父さんは、同じことを言ったよ。
〈歯を磨くように〉
私のお父さんは、歯を磨くように言ったよ。

 1. 毎日磨くように
 2. 歯のケアをするように
 3. ジャンクフードを食べないように
 4. キャンディを食べないように
 5. 栄養のあるものを食べるように
 6. フッ素配合の歯磨きを使うように
 7. あなたが言ったのと同じことを
 8. 磨いてフロッシングするように
 9. りんごを食べるように
10. 毎日フロッシングするように
11. 歯医者に行くように
12. 歯医者の言うことを聞くように

Chapter 9

A small child's first visit with the hygienist
Part V: Fluoride treatment

What is Fluoride?

The topical fluoride treatment is done after the teeth have been thoroughly cleaned. The following is an explanation to the child of how it will be done and why.

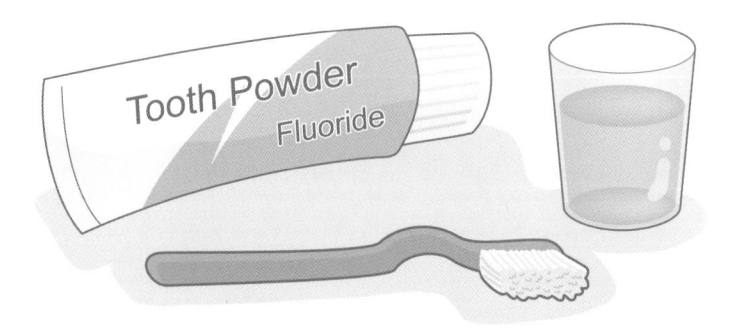

第 9 章

小さな子どもが初めて歯科衛生士と接する時
V．フッ素の応用

フッ素って何？

　フッ素の歯面塗布は、歯を完全にきれいにしてから行われる。以下の対話は、それがどのようにして、またなぜ行われるか子どもに説明するものである。

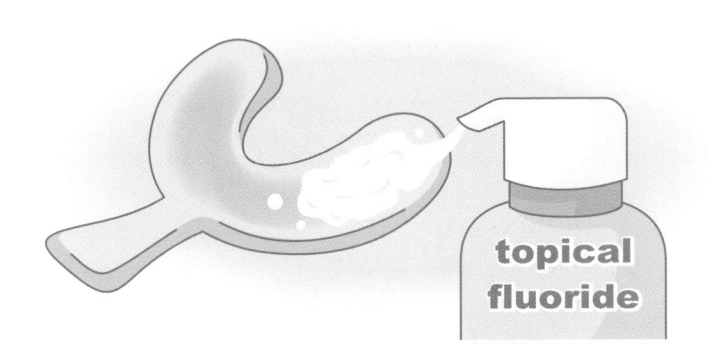

Situation: A continuation of the previous dialogue.

Ms. Kano (dental hygienist): Now that your teeth are clean, we will put some fluoride on them to make them strong.

Bobby: What is fluoride?

Ms. Kano: It is a kind of medicine which makes the teeth strong to help prevent tooth decay.

Bobby: Does it hurt?

Ms. Kano: No, it doesn't hurt at all. All I do is place some fluoride on this sponge and hold it in your mouth for four minutes.

Bobby: Is that all?

Ms. Kano: Yes, that's all. But you should not drink or eat anything for thirty minutes after this treatment.

Bobby: Well, I don't know if I can do that or not. I like to eat.

Ms. Kano: I think that you can go without eating for thirty minutes. Then your teeth will be good and strong.

Bobby: O.K. I'll try not to eat or drink for thirty minutes.

場面：前章の対話の続き。

加納さん（歯科衛生士）：もうあなたの歯がきれいになったから、フッ素を塗って歯を強くしましょう。
ボビー：フッ素って何？
　加納：それは薬の一種で、歯を強くしてむし歯を防ぐのを助けるものよ。
ボビー：痛い？
　加納：いいえ。ぜんぜん痛くないわ。私がするのは、フッ素を少しこのスポンジにつけて、4分間あなたの口の中に入れておくだけよ。
ボビー：それだけ？
　加納：ええ。それだけ。でもこの治療の後30分間は何も飲んだり食べたりしてはいけません。
ボビー：ううん……そんなことできるかどうかわからないなぁ。僕、食べたいよ。
　加納：30分間は食べないでいられると思うわ。そうしたら、あなたの歯は丈夫で強くなりますよ。
ボビー：オーケー　30分間食べたり飲んだりしないようにするよ。

Exercises

I. Substitute the following expressions in the example sentence.

Fluoride is a kind of medicine.
⟨amalgam/restorative material⟩
Amalgam is a kind of restorative material.

1. resin/restorative material
2. lidocaine/anesthetic
3. reversible hydrocolloid/impression material
4. a pedodontist/dentist
5. penicillin/antibiotic
6. composite resin/restorative material
7. aspirin/pain killer
8. gold/precious metal
9. a periodontist/dentist
10. toothbrush/oral hygiene aid
11. toothpick/oral hygiene aid
12. floss/oral hygiene aid

II. Substitute the following expressions in the example sentence.

Fluoride helps prevent tooth decay.
⟨dental disease⟩
Fluoride helps prevent dental disease.

練習問題

Ⅰ．例文の下線部を以下の語句に置き換えなさい。

フッ素は薬の一種です。
〈アマルガム／修復材〉
アマルガムは修復材の一種です。

1. レジン／修復材
2. リドカイン／麻酔
3. 可逆性ハイドロコロイド／印象材
4. 小児歯科医／歯医者
5. ペニシリン／抗生物質
6. コンポジットレジン／修復材
7. アスピリン／痛みどめ
8. 金／貴金属
9. 歯周病専門医／歯医者
10. 歯ブラシ／口腔衛生器具
11. つまようじ／口腔衛生器具
12. フロス／口腔衛生器具

Ⅱ．例文の下線部を以下の語句に置き換えなさい。

フッ素はむし歯を防ぐのを助ける。
〈歯の病気〉
フッ素は歯の病気を防ぐのを助ける。

1. dental problems
2. cavities in your teeth
3. problems
4. dental caries
5. future dental bills
6. decay
7. the need for fillings
8. weak teeth
9. interproximal caries
10. breakdown of the teeth
11. loss of teeth
12. the need for dental treatment

Ⅲ. Substitute the following expressions in the example dialogue.

- Does it <u>hurt</u>?
- No, it doesn't <u>hurt</u> at all.

⟨taste bad⟩
- Does it <u>taste bad</u>?
- No, it doesn't <u>taste bad</u> at all.

1. look bad
2. have a bad odor
3. hurt the teeth
4. hurt the gums
5. stain the teeth
6. stain the gums

1. 歯科の問題
2. むし歯
3. 問題
4. 歯のう蝕
5. これからの歯科治療費
6. むし歯
7. 充填の必要性
8. 弱い歯になる（のを）
9. 歯間のう蝕
10. 歯が割れること
11. 歯を失うこと
12. 歯科治療が必要になる（のを）

Ⅲ．例にあげた対話の下線部を以下の語句に置き換えなさい。

－<u>痛い</u>ですか？
－いいえ、ぜんぜん<u>痛く</u>ありません。
〈いやな味がする〉
－いやな味がしますか？
－いいえ、ぜんぜん<u>いやな味は</u>しません。

1. ひどく見える
2. いやなにおいがある
3. 歯を傷つける
4. 歯ぐきを傷つける
5. 歯にステインをつける
6. 歯ぐきにステインをつける

7. cause problems
8. cause tooth decay
9. take a lot of time
10. restrict movement
11. interfere with function
12. cause brown stains

Ⅳ. Substitute the following expressions in the example dialogue.

- Is it difficult?
- No, it's not difficult at all.
〈easy〉
- Is it easy?
- No, it's not easy at all.

1. large
2. hard
3. light
4. heavy
5. stained
6. decayed
7. a problem
8. a good idea
9. a bad idea
10. rough
11. broken down
12. acceptable

7. 問題の原因になる
8. むし歯の原因になる
9. たくさんの時間がかかる
10. 動きを制限する
11. 機能を妨げる
12. 茶色のステインの原因になる

Ⅳ．例にあげた対話の下線部を以下の語句に置き換えなさい。

－難しいですか？
－いいえ、ぜんぜん難しくありません。
〈簡単だ〉
－簡単ですか？
－いいえ、ぜんぜん簡単ではありません。

1. 大きい
2. 固い
3. 明るい
4. 重い
5. ステインがついている
6. むし歯になっている
7. 問題だ
8. 良い考えだ
9. 悪い考えだ
10. ざらざらしている
11. 壊れている
12. 好ましい

Ⅴ. Substitute the following expressions in the example sentence.

I'll try not to <u>eat</u> for thirty minutes.
⟨talk⟩
I'll try not to <u>talk</u> for thirty minutes.

1. drink water
2. eat snacks
3. eat anything
4. eat candy
5. drink cola
6. drink juices
7. eat or drink
8. forget your instructions
9. complain
10. eat junk food
11. eat a candy bar
12. eat sugar

Ⅴ．例文の下線部を以下の語句に置き換えなさい。

30分間食べないようにします。
〈話す〉
30分間話さないようにします。

1. 水を飲む
2. お菓子を食べる
3. 食べる
4. キャンディを食べる
5. コーラを飲む
6. ジュースを飲む
7. 食べたり飲んだりする
8. 指導を忘れる
9. 文句を言う
10. ジャンクフードを食べる
11. キャンディバーを食べる
12. 砂糖を食べる

Chapter 10

The health history

Are You in Good Health?

Sometimes the hygienist may be requested to take the patient's health history. It is important to record any medicines the patient is taking and to learn if he has had any serious diseases. Be sure to ask the patient if he has any allergies to medicines or dental anesthetics.

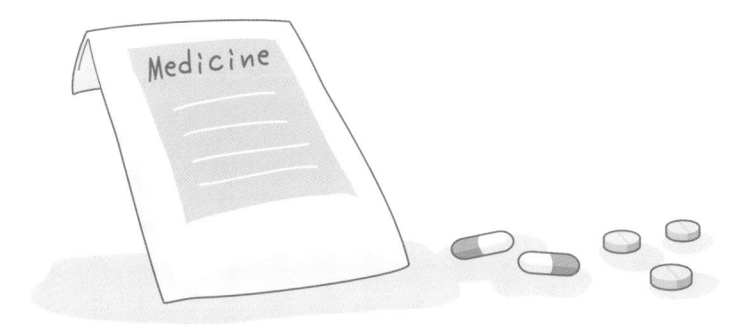

第 10 章

既往歴

健康状態はよいですか？

　時には、歯科衛生士が患者の既往歴を取るように頼まれるかもしれない。患者が飲んでいる薬を記録し、重い病気になったことがあるかどうか知ることが大切である。患者には、必ず、薬や歯科麻酔に対するアレルギーがあるか尋ねなければならない。

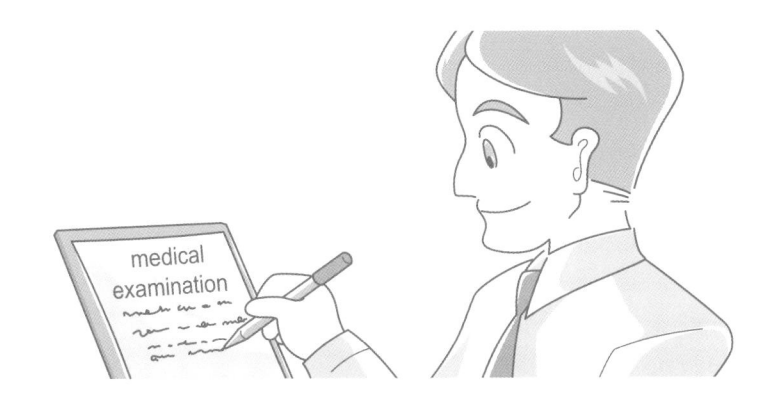

Situation: The dental hygienist is taking the health history of Mr. Collins, a thirty-eight year-old Canadian.

Ms. Hirano (dental hygienist): The doctor has asked me to take your health history.

Mr. Collins: Fine.

Ms. Hirano: Are you in good health?

Mr. Collins: As far as I know.

Ms. Hirano: Are you taking any medication or receiving any medical treatment at this time?

Mr. Collins: Yes. I am taking Inderal.

Ms. Hirano: Could you spell that please?

Mr. Collins: I – N – D – E – R – A – L.

Ms. Hirano: Do you have any allergies to foods or medicines?

Mr. Collins: Not that I know of.

Ms. Hirano: Have you ever had a bad reaction to dental anesthetics?

Mr. Collins: No.

Ms. Hirano: Have you ever had any serious diseases such as tuberculosis, hepatitis, or diabetes?

Mr. Collins: No, I haven't.

Ms. Hirano: When was your last dental checkup?

Mr. Collins: I can't remember exactly, but I think that it was about two years ago.

Ms. Hirano: Is there any other information that we should know about your health history?

Mr. Collins: I don't think so.

場面：歯科衛生士が、38歳のカナダ人、コリンズ氏の既往歴を取っている。

平野さん（歯科衛生士）：先生が私に、既往歴を取ってほしいと言われました。
コリンズ氏：わかりました。
　　平野：健康状態は良いですか？
コリンズ氏：私の知る限りでは、良いです。
　　平野：現在何か薬を飲んだり、または、治療を受けていらっしゃいますか？
コリンズ氏：ええ。Inderalをのんでいます。
　　平野：綴りを教えていただけますか？
コリンズ氏：I-N-D-E-R-A-L
　　平野：食べ物や薬に何かアレルギーはありますか？
コリンズ氏：私の知る限りではありません。
　　平野：歯科麻酔に悪い反応があったことがありますか？
コリンズ氏：いいえ。
　　平野：結核、肝炎、糖尿病などのような、重い病気になったことはありますか？
コリンズ氏：いいえ、ありません。
　　平野：最後に歯科のチェックを受けられたのはいつですか？
コリンズ氏：はっきりとは覚えていませんが、あれは2年ぐらい前だったと思います。
　　平野：あなたの既往歴に関して、私共が知っておくべきことは他にありますか？
コリンズ氏：ないと思います。

Exercises

I. Substitute the following expressions in the example sentence.

The hygienist may be requested to <u>take the patient's health history</u>.
⟨give flossing instructions⟩
The hygienist may be requested to <u>give flossing instructions</u>.

1. give brushing instructions
2. do an oral prophylaxis
3. do nutrition counseling
4. help the patient
5. do a fluoride treatment
6. clean the patient's teeth
7. explain dental treatment to the patient
8. work as a dental assistant
9. record all medications that the patient uses
10. take the patient's blood pressure
11. polish the teeth
12. review the medical history

II. Substitute the following expressions in the example dialogue.

−Have you ever had <u>diabetes</u>?
−No, I haven't.
⟨hepatitis⟩

練習問題

Ⅰ．例文の下線部を以下の語句に置き換えなさい。

歯科衛生士が患者の既往歴を取るように頼まれるかもしれない。

〈フロッシング指導をする〉
歯科衛生士がフロッシング指導をするように頼まれるかもしれない。

1. ブラッシング指導をする
2. 口腔清掃をする
3. 栄養カウンセリングをする
4. 患者を手伝う
5. フッ素を応用する
6. 患者の歯をきれいにする
7. 患者に歯科治療の説明をする
8. 歯科助手として働く
9. 患者が使っているすべての薬を記録する
10. 患者の血圧を計る
11. 歯を研磨する
12. 既往歴を調べる

Ⅱ．例にあげた対話の下線部を以下の語句に置き換えなさい。

－糖尿病になったことがありますか？
－いいえ、ありません。
〈肝炎〉

― Have you ever had hepatitis?
― No, I haven't.

1. a serious disease
2. tuberculosis
3. an unusual reaction to medicines
4. heart trouble
5. epilepsy
6. anemia
7. rheumatic fever
8. venereal disease
9. asthma
10. high blood pressure
11. kidney disease
12. an unusual reaction to dental anesthetics

Ⅲ. Substitute the following expressions in the example sentence.

She came to the clinic because of gingival bleeding.
〈because of a toothache〉
She came to the clinic because of a toothache.

1. because of pain
2. because of bad breath
3. for a checkup
4. for a cleaning
5. because she likes the dentist

－肝炎になったことがありますか？
－いいえ、ありません。

1. 重い病気
2. 結核
3. 薬に対する異常な反応
4. 心臓病
5. てんかん
6. 貧血
7. リウマチ熱
8. 性病
9. ぜんそく
10. 高血圧
11. 腎臓病
12. 歯科麻酔に対する異常な反応

Ⅲ．例文の下線部を以下の語句に置き換えなさい。

彼女は、歯肉出血のため、診療所に来た。
〈歯痛のため〉
彼女は、歯痛のため、診療所に来た。

1. 痛みのため
2. 口臭のため
3. 検診のため
4. クリーニングのため
5. 歯医者が好きなので

6. because she does not want to get gum disease
7. because of poor oral health
8. for oral hygiene instructions
9. for a radiographic examination
10. for a diagnosis
11. for a second opinion
12. for an amalgam filling

Ⅳ. Substitute the following expressions in the example sentence.

The doctor has asked me to take the patient's health history.
⟨give flossing instructions⟩
The doctor has asked me to give flossing instructions.

1. give brushing and flossing instructions
2. do a cleaning
3. discuss nutrition
4. help you floss
5. put fluoride on the teeth
6. clean your teeth
7. explain the treatment
8. work as an assistant
9. help the receptionist
10. take your blood pressure
11. polish your teeth
12. review the health history

6. 歯ぐきの病気になりたくないので
7. 口腔が健康でないので
8. 口腔衛生指導のため
9. エックス線写真検査のため
10. 診断をしてもらうため
11. 第2の（医者の）意見を聞くために
12. アマルガム充填のため

Ⅳ．例文の下線部を以下の語句に置き換えなさい。

先生が私に、患者の既往歴を取るように頼みました。
〈フロス指導をする〉
先生が私に、フロス指導をするように頼みました。

1. 歯ブラシ指導とフロス指導をする
2. クリーニングをする
3. 栄養について話す
4. フロスするのを手伝う
5. 歯にフッ素を塗布する
6. あなたの歯をクリーニングする
7. 治療について説明する
8. 助手として働く
9. 受付の人を手伝う
10. あなたの血圧を計る
11. あなたの歯を研磨する
12. 既往歴を調べる

V. Substitute the following expressions in the example sentence.

Ask if the patient has had diabetes.
⟨hepatitis⟩
Ask if the patient has had hepatitis.

1. bleeding disorders
2. cancer
3. an unusual reaction to antibiotics
4. heart problems
5. arthritis
6. anemia
7. rheumatic fever
8. extensive dental treatment
9. asthma
10. high blood pressure
11. liver problems
12. an unusual reaction to medicines

Ⅴ．例文の下線部を以下の語句に置き換えなさい。

患者が糖尿病になったことがあるかどうか尋ねなさい。
〈肝炎〉
患者が肝炎になったことがあるかどうか尋ねなさい。

1. 出血異常
2. 癌
3. 抗生物質に対する異常な反応
4. 心臓の問題
5. 関節炎
6. 貧血
7. リウマチ熱
8. 広範囲にわたる歯科治療
9. ぜんそく
10. 高血圧
11. 肝臓の問題
12. 薬に対する異常な反応

付録

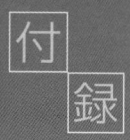

患者とのコミュニケーションで役立つ最重要用語100語

以下は、歯科衛生士と患者とのコミュニケーションに役立つ最重要用語100語を、アルファベット順に並べたものである。これらは特に歯科用語を知らない人にもわかる言葉である。

A

ache	痛む、痛み
adjust	合わせる、調整する
allergy	アレルギー
amalgam	アマルガム
anesthetic	麻酔薬
antibiotics	抗生物質
appointment	予約、アポイント、約束
aspirin	アスピリン
assistant	（歯科）助手

B

bad breath	口臭
bleed	出血する
braces	矯正装置
bridge	加工義歯

C

calculus	歯石
cavity	むし歯、窩洞
cement	セメント
checkup	（歯科）検診
cheek	頬
clean	（歯を）清掃する
cleaning	（歯の）清掃
clinic	診療所
comfortable	楽な
crown	歯冠、クラウン

D

debris	残遺物、汚物
decay	むし歯
dental	歯科の、歯の
dentist	歯科医

dentistry	歯科医学	**J**	
denture	義歯	junk food	ジャンクフード（栄養がない食品）
diagnosis	診断		
discomfort	不快		
E		**L**	
emergency	緊急	lip	唇
examination	予診、診査	lower teeth	下顎の歯
examine	診察する	**M**	
extract	抜く	medicine	薬
		molar	臼歯
F		**N**	
filling	充填（物）	nervous	神経の
fit	適合する		
floss	フロス、糸	**O**	
flossing	フロッシング	operation	手術、処置
fluoride	フッ素	oral	口腔の
G		oral prophylaxis	口腔清掃
gums	歯ぐき	orthodontic	歯科矯正の
		orthodontics	歯科矯正学
H		**P**	
health	健康	pain	痛み
hygienist	衛生士	pain killer	鎮痛剤
		patient	患者
I		pedodontist	小児歯科医
impression	印象	penicillin	ペニシリン
inflamed	炎症性の	periodontal	歯周の
inflammation	炎症	permanent teeth	永久歯
inlay	インレー		

0141

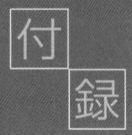

plaque	プラーク		**T**	
polish	研磨する	temporary	暫間の
porcelain	ポーセレン、陶材	tenderness	触痛
prepare	形成する、準備する	tongue	舌
primary teeth	乳歯	toothache	歯痛
		toothbrush	歯ブラシ
R		toothpaste	歯磨剤
recall	呼び戻す、リコール	treat	治療する、処置する
receptionist	受付係	treatment	治療、処置
restore	修復する	treatment plan	治療計画
rinse	ゆすぐ		
root canal treatment	根管治療	**U**	
rubber dam	ラバーダム	uncomfortable	不愉快な
		upper teeth	上顎の歯
S			
saliva	唾液	**W**	
scaler	スケーラー	waiting room	待合室
sealants	シーラント	wisdom tooth	智歯
sensitive	敏感な		
sensitivity	敏感	**X**	
specialist	専門医	X-ray	エックス線
stain	有色性沈着物、着色		
surgery	外科学、外科		
swelling	腫脹		
swollen	腫れ上がった		

メモ

メモ

クインテッセンス出版の書籍・雑誌は，歯学書専用通販サイト『歯学書.COM』にてご購入いただけます．

PCからのアクセスは…
歯学書　検索

携帯電話からのアクセスは…
QRコードからモバイルサイトへ

QUINTESSENCE PUBLISHING
日本

改訂版　クインテッセンス歯科英会話シリーズ
PART2 英語が話せる歯科衛生士！

1989年8月25日　第1版第1刷発行
2007年9月10日　第2版第1刷発行
2019年1月25日　第2版第2刷発行

著　者　Thomas R. Ward
　　　　（トーマス　アール　ウォード）

発行人　北峯康充

発行所　クインテッセンス出版株式会社
　　　　東京都文京区本郷3丁目2番6号　〒113-0033
　　　　クイントハウスビル　電話(03)5842-2270(代表)
　　　　　　　　　　　　　　　(03)5842-2272(営業部)
　　　　　　　　　　　　　　　(03)5842-2279(編集部)
　　　　web page address　https://www.quint-j.co.jp/

印刷・製本　サン美術印刷株式会社

Ⓒ2007　クインテッセンス出版株式会社　　　　禁無断転載・複写
Printed in Japan　　　　　　　　　　　　　　落丁本・乱丁本はお取り替えします
ISBN978-4-87417-972-7　C3047　　　　　　　定価はカバーに表示してあります